Evaluating the Treatment of Drug Abuse in the European Union

Papers arising from an EMCDDA workshop held in Athens, Greece, on 17–18 March 1997

PLANNING GROUP

Margareta Nilson
Anna Kokkevi
Petra Paula Merino
Monica Blum

EDITORIAL GROUP

Oswin Baker
Jane Mounteney

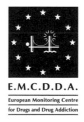

E.M.C.D.D.A.
European Monitoring Centre
for Drugs and Drug Addiction

A great deal of additional information on the European Union is available on the Internet. It can be accessed through the Europa server (http://europa.eu.int)

Information about the European Monitoring Centre for Drugs and Drug Addiction is available at **http://www.emcdda.org**

Cataloguing data can be found at the end of this publication

Luxembourg: Office for Official Publications of the European Communities, 1999

ISBN 92-9168-051-6

Printed in Italy

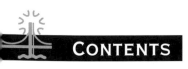

CONTENTS

ACKNOWLEDGEMENTS

*T*his monograph contains the papers presented at the 'Workshop on the Evaluation of Drug Abuse Treatment' held in Athens from 17–18 March 1997. The volume highlights the work of the University Mental Health Research Institute (UMHRI) in Athens – and particularly of Anna Kokkevi – in organising the workshop on behalf of the EMCDDA.

Thanks are due to the workshop speakers, and to Oswin Baker and Jane Mounteney of the Institute for the Study of Drug Dependence (ISDD) in London who edited them into a coherent whole.

Thanks also go to the staff of the EMCDDA, in particular to Margareta Nilson, Petra Paula Merino, Rachel Neaman and Monica Blum, for their work on the workshop and this monograph.

Georges Estievenart
Director
EMCDDA

GENERAL INTRODUCTION

GENERAL INTRODUCTION

Margareta Nilson

The mandate of the European Monitoring Centre for Drugs and Drug Addiction (EMCDDA), as set out in its founding Regulation, is to collect, analyse and disseminate objective, reliable and comparable information on drugs and drug addiction in the European Union (EU).[1] One of the EMCDDA's primary areas of focus is the demand for drugs and reducing that demand.

Treating drug addiction is one of the main pillars of drug demand reduction. In all 15 EU Member States, specific treatment systems have developed over the last few decades. In recent years, moreover, many of these systems have been revised and diversified, largely in response to the spread of HIV and AIDS and to increasing financial restraints in the public sector.

Knowledge about the actual effects of treatment – what works – has not, however, always kept pace with these developments. As a result, it is essential to develop and disseminate high-quality information about appropriate methods, instruments and indicators to enhance the comprehensive evaluation of treatment programmes for drug users, as well as to allow for comparative evaluation of different programmes. Such knowledge not only enables policy-makers to make informed and appropriate decisions, but also increases the quality of the work carried out by all those involved in the drugs field. Furthermore, high-quality information can only be obtained from evaluated treatments.

The EMCDDA is, therefore, focusing on promoting the evaluation of drug treatment and disseminating this information to policy-makers and professionals throughout Europe.

The starting point for this work was the EMCDDA 'Workshop on the Evaluation of Drug Abuse Treatment', held in Athens from 17–18 March 1997. The main aims of this meeting were:

- to function as a forum for exchanging ideas and experiences;
- to define the EMCDDA's mid-term Work Programme in the field of treatment evaluation; and
- to raise the profile of the EMCDDA within the relevant scientific community in Europe.

The participants were asked to tackle priority issues in treatment evaluation, such as the conceptual frameworks of evaluation and treatment, and the aims of assessing treatment. Methodologies and implementation were also targeted, as were ways of

---

[1] European Council Regulation (EEC) no. 302/93, 8 February 1993.

making evaluation information more relevant to professionals and decision-makers and promoting communication between all those involved.

The workshop was attended by experts from Germany, Greece, Italy, the Netherlands, Sweden and the United Kingdom. The COST-A6 working group on evaluating treatment and the World Health Organisation (WHO)'s Programme on Substance Abuse were also represented.[2] The two-day meeting began by examining the main areas of treatment evaluation. This was followed by a debate, and recommendations for further action were then made to the EMCDDA.

This monograph is made up of the papers presented at the workshop, and is divided into three sections:

- the theory of treatment evaluation;
- the practice of treatment evaluation; and
- the policy of treatment evaluation.

These sections are followed by a workshop summary, a list of the recommendations made to the EMCDDA for its mid-term work plan on treatment evaluation and latest perspectives on the Centre's work in this field.

---

[2] COST A-6 is a programme run by the European Commission's Directorate General XII (Science, Research, Development) to gain valid information concerning the impact of various drug policies and measures on the extent, nature and consequences of drug abuse.

THE THEORY OF DRUG-TREATMENT EVALUATION

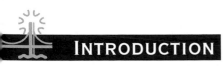

PART I

INTRODUCTION

*I*n Chapter 1, Vincent Hendriks looks at the current state of treatment evaluation. He argues that evaluators, researchers and practitioners are still faced with
the same questions as 20 or 30 years ago, including: does treatment work?
What constitutes 'treatment' and 'success'? What are the 'active ingredients' of treatment? And what treatment works for which client? Hendriks goes on to explore the
difficult research issue of randomisation and seeks a way through the ethical tangle
by discussing 'client, treatment and process'.

Chapter 2, by Petra Paula Merino of the EMCDDA, presents an overview of the
treatment-evaluation literature, highlighting prominent themes and dilemmas
including the non-comparability of research findings and the problems of defining
effectiveness. Merino discusses how few investigations specifically examine the way
staffing and working conditions relate to the effectiveness of treatment and how the
study of treatment has often been divorced from that of the drug user.

In Chapter 3, Mats Fridell examines some of the most complex areas in the evaluation of residential treatment. He demonstrates that an array of different research
approaches must be considered, depending on whether the aim is to study effects,
outcome or quality. No single research design provides the answers to all these
fields, and many – if not most – of the problems related to institutional treatment
might be better approached by models other than the traditional randomised control
study.

Chapter 4 examines the methodological aspects of evaluation in greater detail, in particular the randomised control study itself. While arguing that such studies provide
the best chance for valid evaluation, Fabio Mariani identifies a number of issues
which make randomised controls difficult in reality. One of these problems is the low
level of statistical and epidemiological competence among drug professionals,
and he calls on the EMCDDA to encourage greater knowledge of such matters.

In Chapter 5, Evi Hatziandreou introduces and defines the contemporary issue of
economic evaluation – a form of research that identifies, measures, values and
compares the costs and benefits of different approaches to treatment. As such, she
argues, economic evaluation deals explicitly with choices by examining the consequences of any intervention under consideration. Hatziandreou outlines economic
evaluation methods, presents the results of such techniques and recommends ways
of realising the full potential of this form of assessment.

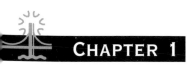

EVALUATING DRUG-ABUSE TREATMENT: CURRENT AND FUTURE PERSPECTIVES

Vincent Hendriks

Over the past three decades, an enormous amount of research has been conducted on evaluating the treatment of addiction. Evaluation studies range from the large-scale US Drug Abuse Reporting Program (DARP) and Treatment Outcome Prospective Study (TOPS) initiatives of the 1960s and 1970s, and the current National Treatment Outcome Research Study (NTORS) in the UK, to numerous smaller-scale clinical investigations, often at individual programme level.

Despite these considerable efforts, addiction-treatment researchers in the 1990s – and into the next millennium – are and still will be confronted with very much the same core questions as those of 20 or 30 years ago. These questions include:

- Does treatment work and what constitutes 'treatment' and 'success'?
- How does treatment work and what are its active ingredients?
- What kind of treatment works for what kind of client?

This chapter provides some answers to these perennial and fundamental questions.

Does treatment work and what constitutes 'treatment' and 'success'?

Many studies have indicated that treatment 'works' for a considerable number of clients. Roughly speaking, the 'rule of thirds' (Miller and Sanchez-Craig, 1996) seems to apply to treatment outcome for both alcoholism and illicit drug use: about one-third of clients become abstinent; one-third improve, but are not abstinent; and one-third do not improve following treatment.

While there is cumulative evidence that treatment does 'work', it is also clear that most of that evidence comes from naturalistic studies that have used a wide variety of methods to evaluate treatment outcome. Just how easy it is for different approaches to lead to different results is shown by Miller and Sanchez-Craig (1996), who gave the following advice to treatment programmes faced with increasing pressure from funders to show high success rates:

- choose only cases with good prognoses to evaluate;
- keep follow-up periods as short as possible;

- avoid control or comparison groups;
- choose outcome measures carefully;
- focus only on alcohol or drug variables;
- use liberal definitions of success;
- rely exclusively on self-report; and
- always declare victory, regardless of the findings!

If all these recommendations are followed, Miller and Sanchez-Craig guarantee that success rates can double, triple or even quadruple, boosting them from a meagre 20–30% to 80% and over.

The issue of randomisation

While Miller and Sanchez-Craig may be poking fun at the field, many of their 'recommendations' – particularly the third ('avoid control or comparison groups') – are widely followed. Although, in the short term, this may ease the pressure from funding organisations, in the long term, it is likely to have negative consequences for the validity of treatment evaluation and of treatments themselves.

Problems related to lack of randomisation

Because of practical and ethical constraints, clients have rarely been randomised into treatment and non-treatment samples, or even into groups under different treatment conditions. The bulk of evaluation studies either examine only one form of treatment (without any control or comparison) or look at different programmes in which clients are self-selected. Typically, the effect of the treatment is then determined by comparing pre- with post-treatment behaviours.

Obviously, applying non-controlled designs severely limits the reliability of the conclusions that can be drawn. Without randomisation, it is impossible to tell whether the observed change is truly an effect of treatment or of something else. In such situations, many confounding factors are free to exert their influence:

- Although the moment of admission to treatment is by no means accidental (being related to an upsurge in an individual's severe problems), the moment of follow-up is usually determined by the researcher. Purely on the basis of this difference, less problematic behaviour is likely at the time of follow-up.

- Clients may over-exaggerate their problematic behaviour at intake, in order to convince the treatment staff of their need for help.

- Conversely, clients may under-represent their problems at the time of follow-up, in order to reduce possible cognitive dissonance. In particular, this may be the case when the client has attended an intensive, long-term treatment programme with little or no success.

- In addition, under-reporting of problems at follow-up may be related to the client's wish to satisfy the therapist or treatment staff (the so-called 'hello–goodbye' effect).

- Clients may assign different meanings to their problems during and after treatment (the 'response shift'). For example, they may view their problems as less severe because they have been confronted with other clients who have worse problems.

As well as the lack of randomised control, the validity of outcome results may be threatened by a host of other factors, many of them already reflected in the 'advice' given by Miller and Sanchez-Craig. Two practical factors – which nearly every researcher in the addiction field has been faced with – deserve special mention:

- *High drop-out rates during treatment:* typically the highest drop-out rates occur in the early weeks of treatment and then decline.

- *Low and selective response rates at follow-up:* when using a longer follow-up period, non-response rates of over 50% are not uncommon. Non-respondents generally evidence more problems than respondents and are more likely to have unorthodox lifestyles.

Problems related to randomisation

Given the serious threats to the validity of outcome results caused by the lack of randomisation, why is this method not applied more often in the addiction field? Three major problems affect the application of a randomised control design in naturalistic treatment research (De Leon *et al.*, 1994a):

- *Ethical constraints:* assignment to a 'no-treatment' condition, or to a 'more-versus-less' treatment condition, actually means withholding services.

- *Practical constraints:* clients in the 'no-treatment' group may seek treatment elsewhere or may be referred to other programmes by family or courts, thereby causing research 'contamination' and 'within-group variance' in the 'no-treatment' control group. There are often high drop-out rates in the 'no-treatment' group prior to the start of the study (due to 'frustration bias'). This seriously breaches the requirement or assumption in randomised assignment that client-groups are comparable at baseline.

- *Logical flaws:* in real life, clients often prefer a particular kind of treatment, which is reflected in the way they select one or another programme. The effect of treatment at least partly depends on the client's readiness to engage in a specific form of it, and so – paradoxically – self-selection represents a prerequisite for treatment effectiveness rather than a problem.

Randomisation into different modalities or programmes may mitigate these differences in preference, but it also causes much 'within-group variance' as a result of client–treatment mismatches regarding motivation and readiness.

Although mismatches may be randomly distributed between the two groups, the effect on the client may differ substantially (De Leon *et al.*, 1994a). For example, the effect of a mismatch on a young client with a short addiction history and stable social environment who is randomised into a long-term therapeutic community is likely to be much greater than that on an older client with a long history of opiate use who is randomised into a methadone-maintenance programme.

Hence, both randomisation and its lack may seriously threaten the validity of outcome results in naturalistic studies. To find a solution to these problems, two alternative approaches have been suggested:

- to apply non-randomised designs, providing an opportunity to compensate for the loss of 'power' of the randomised approach by incorporating into the evaluation information not only on the client, but also on the treatment and its process; or
- to restrict randomisation to specific components *within* a treatment.

The major problem encountered in both approaches, however, is that treatment is still very much a 'black box', and that neither treatment as a whole, nor the interventions within treatment, are well described or understood.

How does treatment work?

The questions of how treatment works, what are its active ingredients and what works for what kind of client can be approached from the following general regression model (Ball and Ross, 1991; De Leon *et al.*, 1994b):

$$\text{Outcome} = \text{constant} + \text{client} + \text{treatment} + \text{process} + \text{error}$$

This model holds that treatment outcome is a function of a constant (people can change without treatment), a variety of client characteristics (demographic background, drug-use history, psychological status, etc.), treatment factors (type of treatment, treatment goal, etc.), process variables (intensity and duration of the intervention received by the client) and an error component (measurement error). With this general model as a background, the two approaches described above (non-randomised and restricted randomisation) can be summarised as follows.

Non-randomised approach

This first approach aims to explore the relative contribution to treatment outcome of client characteristics and of those components related to the programme and process in a naturalistic design.

Instead of *controlling* the influence of client differences through randomisation, this approach aims explicitly to trace those influences and to explore the interaction of client, treatment programme and process on outcome. Clients clearly vary in many respects and attend different treatments and follow divergent paths regarding the type of intervention received and its duration. Treatment outcome can therefore be measured by classifying these client–treatment trajectories, and by comparing the changes during and after treatment across the subgroups.

Restricted randomisation

The second approach can be applied to subsequent investigations of the effectiveness of specific treatment components (such as cue exposure) by means of randomised trials *within* the treatment under investigation. As mentioned above, the main problem with randomising clients into different treatments is that they nearly always have a preference for a certain type of programme (therapeutic community, detoxification, methadone maintenance, etc.). This preference does not exist to such an extent at the level of specific therapeutic components within a treatment, thus making controlled randomised trials feasible. Trials can be made using existing treatment components, but also by adding new components to 'treatment as usual'.

To summarise, while the first approach aims to explore the contribution to treatment outcome of a full range of components on specific groups of clients, the second approach pinpoints the contribution to treatment outcome of a specific component on a full range of clients.

While conceptually sensible, it is clear that the usefulness of the general model of the first approach ('exploration') depends on the ability to 'fill in' each of the boxes (client, treatment and process), and that – on the technical level – the practical application of this model depends on the use of quite complex multivariate regression techniques.

Client, treatment, process

Although a great deal of progress has been made in measuring client characteristics reliably, virtually no attempt has been made to study treatment or process variables, and no reliable and valid instruments exist to measure them.

This bears directly on the so-called 'matching hypothesis', which states that some types of treatment or intervention are better suited to certain types of client than other treatments. According to McLellan and Alterman (1991), the lack of empirical support for the matching hypothesis may be mainly due to the lack of a reliable, valid, practical and generalisable instrument to measure treatment interventions. Clearly, in order to match clients to treatments and to investigate the effectiveness of this matching, sufficient information is needed about both the client and the treatment. In terms of the general regression model, this means that the relevant variables in each of the model's boxes have to be identified and quantified using measurement instruments.

The client

Much progress has been made in measuring a wide range of client characteristics. Since the 1980s, there has been a shift towards a multidimensional assessment of functioning in various life areas (including health, substance use and psychology). This has been coupled with a move towards using standardised instruments, such as the Addiction Severity Index (ASI – McLellan *et al.*, 1980) and the Opiate Treatment Index (Darke *et al.*, 1992), all of which can be used for both research and diagnostic or screening purposes.

Despite these developments, however, client factors have rarely been found to explain more than 15–20% of the variance in treatment outcome, thus leaving approximately 80% unexplained. This raises the question of whether the proportion of variance accounted for by client factors can be increased, for example by improving the quality, reliability and validity of measurement, or by widening the range of client variables collected.

As for the reliability and validity of measuring client characteristics, a number of problems still remain. In particular, there are difficulties inherent in 'dual diagnosis', measuring co-existing psychopathology and its relationship to drug use. For example, in practice it is very difficult to distinguish between psychopathology and drug-induced psychiatric symptoms, which may blur the prognostic significance of this factor in treatment. In addition, screening instruments in this area (such as the Symptom Check-List 90 (SCL-90), Personality Diagnostic Questionnaire (PDQ) and ASI) have generally shown high rates of false positives when compared to a categorical psychiatric diagnosis.

Turning to the range of client variables collected, much can still be gained by focusing on the so-called 'treatment-dependent' client variables (Kersten *et al.*, 1995), as well as the 'treatment-independent' variables that are usually collected, such as demographic background, drug-use history and social functioning.

Treatment-dependent client variables

Treatment-dependent client variables only arise in the relationship between client and treatment, and refer to such factors as the type of help needed, the client's motivation for treatment and client expectations. These types of variables are rarely collected, and very few attempts have been made to develop standardised instruments in this area.

According to the (mainly US) literature, three areas of treatment-dependent client variables may be important for prognosis and client–treatment matching. They should thus be considered when developing instruments (see Kersten *et al.*, 1995):

- the client's preference for a specific treatment;
- the client's own 'addiction model'; and
- the client's 'stage of change'.

The client's preference for a specific treatment

This goes back to the self-selecting process described earlier. According to Miller (1989) 'self-matching' is a prerequisite for successful treatment, and should be seen in terms of providing adequate information to the client about his or her treatment options, the content and purpose of the treatment and the likelihood of a positive outcome. Several researchers have found evidence to support the importance of self-matching (Sanchez-Craig, 1980; Thornton *et al.*, 1977).

For the purposes of instrument development, self-selection issues should be explored and data collected on the role played by self-selection in the intake process. For example:

- Does the client have a specific treatment preference?
- Did this preference exist before information was given to the client, or did the preference result from the interaction between the client and intake staff?
- Did the client actually undertake the treatment of choice?

The client's own 'addiction model'

This term refers to the client's general perspective on his or her addiction problems. There are two central questions here (Brickman *et al.*, 1982; Kersten *et al.*, 1995):

- Does the client feel responsible for the causes of his or her addiction?
- Does the client feel responsible for changing his or her addiction?

By similarly categorising treatments according to clients' views of their responsibility for addiction and change, clients may be matched to a treatment bearing the same philosophy. If, for example, the client does not feel responsible either for the causes of, or for changing, the addiction, then a medical treatment employing a disease model may be most appropriate. Several studies support this view (for example, Colon and Massey, 1988; Miller *et al.*, 1993).

The client's 'stage of change'

In 1983, Prochaska and DiClemente postulated their now-familiar model of 'stages of change', which describes the process of achieving abstinence through the various stages of pre-contemplation, contemplation, preparation, action, maintenance and relapse or continued abstinence (Prochaska and DiClemente, 1983).

According to these authors, many studies have demonstrated the significance of 'stage-membership' for treatment prognosis (see Prochaska and Velicer, 1996), but others have challenged this conclusion and argue that strong empirical support for the model is lacking (Davidson, 1992; Farkas *et al.*, 1996). Nevertheless, taken at face value the model has excellent validity and – as a model of *change* – has obvious applications.

Regarding instrument development, several questionnaires have been developed to cover the 'stages-of-change' concept. Prochaska *et al.* (1988), for instance, produced the Processes of Change Questionnaire which measures ten such processes and which has been tested psychometrically in various studies (O'Connor *et al.*, 1996; Prochaska *et al.*, 1988; Velicer *et al.*, 1995).

Several researchers have also developed instruments to measure client motivation for change or for treatment. For example, De Leon and Jainchill (1986) developed

Circumstance, Motivation, Readiness, Suitability (CMRS), and found empirical support for CMRS scores predicting treatment retention (De Leon *et al.*, 1994b). More recently, Miller and Tonigan (1996) developed the States of Change Readiness and Treatment Eagerness Scale (SOCRATES) to measure the client's motivation for change. Given the importance of such motivation, each of these instruments should be examined for application and further development.

Treatment

Studies have rarely involved treatment or process variables in their evaluation model, other than using 'time in treatment' as an intermediate variable or simply describing the main type of treatment under investigation. The fact that 'time in treatment' has consistently been found to be a strong predictor of outcome is an indication (but no more than that) that 'something' happens during treatment. An increase in the duration of treatment, however, should not be confused with having received more treatment, since clients may have received different amounts of treatment during a similar time period. Clients also differ in the amount of time they need to change.

The reason why so many studies have disregarded this area is that it is very difficult to identify and quantify what happens during treatment – either from the client's or from the treatment's perspective.

On a conceptual level, four basic sources of information about the treatment programme and process can be distinguished. These information sources may serve as a starting point for future instrument development, data collection and evaluation research:

Treatment:

- general description of the type of treatment;
- services offered to the client (type, intensity, duration).

Process:

- services received by the client (type, intensity, duration);
- client change during treatment.

General description of the type of treatment

To isolate treatment variables effectively, it is necessary to understand what is actually meant by the term 'treatment'. This entails distinguishing between the main types and sub-types of treatment, and between its modality, goals, planned duration and accessibility. The following example (which has been adapted from the Pompidou Group's Drug Treatment Definitive Protocol) may serve as a framework for such a classification (Hartnoll, 1994):

Table 1: Classification of types of treatment

Types of treatment programme

Specialised residential
- hospital in-patient unit
- therapeutic community
- other (specify)

Specialised outpatient/non-residential
- hospital outpatient treatment centre
- structured day-care centre/day hospital
- local health/social-service centre
- low threshold/drop-in/street agency
- other (specify)

General service-based
- in-patient psychiatric hospital
- outpatient mental-health-care centre
- primary-health-care service
- residential social-care facility
- non-residential social-care facility
- other non-specialised residential (specify)
- other non-specialised non-residential (specify)

Treatment unit in prison

Type of treatment modality
- detoxification/short term reduction
- longer-term drug substitution
- medicament-free therapy/longer-term psychosocial treatment
- advice/counselling/short intervention/support

Goal of treatment
- abstinence
- stabilisation/harm-reduction/secondary prevention
- behavioural change

Planned duration of treatment
- short (<1 month)
- mid-term (1–6 months)
- long (>6 months)

Accessibility of treatment
- waiting list (e.g., average duration previous year)
- insurance coverage (yes/no)
- 'motivation' required (e.g., threshold at intake: low/middle/high; abstinence required)
- planned total duration of treatment (short, middle, long)
- geographical location (urban/suburban/rural)

Services offered to the client

With respect to the second source of treatment information, it is preferable to collect data using the before ('intake') and after ('follow-up') format, as this provides an opportunity to link pre-, during- and post-treatment variables directly.

One way to do so is to adopt a general instrument such as the Addiction Severity Index with its six problem areas, and collect information about the treatment pro- gramme and process in each. For each area, the treatment's active ingredients should be described, as well as the extent to which they were offered to the clients. It should be noted, however, that much qualitative research is still needed to identify and quantify the relevant variables in each problem area. As an example, the domains of therapeutic ingredients and physical health are described in Table 2 below.

Process

There are two sources of process information: services received by the client; and client change during treatment.

Services received by the client

This area of information refers to the treatment elements that were actually received by the individual client during treatment or during a certain treatment period. Parallel to the factors discussed above, each component can be described in terms of the following:

* services actually received by the client: type, frequency, duration
* the result of these interventions: staff-rating
* client satisfaction with these interventions: client-rating

Information on the type, frequency and duration of services actually received by an individual client can be obtained through a treatment-registration system that should be carefully and regularly maintained.

As for the second area of information, staff members who are actively involved with a particular client can be asked regularly to complete a questionnaire in which they rate the client's developments with respect to each of the areas described in the previous section (group therapy, individual therapy, family therapy, results of physical health interventions, etc.). The third area similarly informs the evaluator about the client's satisfaction with each of the interventions described in the previous section.

Client change during treatment

This final area of information is aimed at collecting data – as objectively as possible – about the ways in which the individual client changes during treatment with respect to each of the main areas described above (substance use, psychosocial

Table 2: Therapeutic ingredients and physical health

Therapeutic ingredients:
    Substance use
    Psychosocial

Therapeutic ingredients:	*Offered to clients:*
Personal mentor available	no/yes

Group therapy:
- no/passive/active/standard
- supportive   [type/frequency/duration]
- confrontational
- behavioural
- cue exposure/relapse prevention
- problem-solving/cognitive
- bio-feedback
- other (specify)

Individual therapy:
- no/passive/active/standard
- psycho-analytical   [type/frequency/duration]
- supportive counselling
- behavioural
- cue exposure/relapse prevention
- problem-solving/cognitive
- other (specify)

Family therapy
- no/passive/active/standard   [type/frequency/duration]

Substance-use education
- no/passive/active/standard   [type/frequency/duration]

Self-help (12 steps/NA/AA)
- no/passive/active/standard   [type/frequency/duration]

Medication
- no/passive/active/standard   [type/dosage/frequency/duration]

Additional ingredients:
    Physical health
    Employment/education/housing/financial
    Legal
    Social/family
    Psychiatric

Physical health:	*Offered to clients:*
Physician available	no/yes

Medical screening/check-up at intake
- no/passive/active/standard   [type/referral]

Medical screening/check-up during treatment
- no/passive/active/standard   [type/frequency/referral]

Health education:
- no/passive/active/standard
- general health/hygiene/sports/nutrition   [type/frequency]
- drug-use risk behaviour

functioning, physical health, employment, legal problems, social/family problems and psychiatric problems). At the same time as assessing the client's status at intake, an 'in-treatment' assessment can be conducted, using an instrument similar to that at intake and focusing on the client's situation during, for example, the previous month.

The role of the EMCDDA

When discussing the potential role of the European Monitoring Centre for Drugs and Drug Addiction in evaluating substance-use treatment in Europe, three aspects stand out:

- the many difficulties involved in improving the general methodology of evaluation studies;

- the multitude of problems associated with identifying key variables and developing instruments, in particular in – but not limited to – the areas of treatment and process variables; and

- the current low level of compatibility in data collection and evaluation methods within and between European Member states.

It should be apparent from this chapter that there is an inherent friction between improvements in the first two areas and improvement in the third. Greater compatibility is often sacrificed to further refinements in data collection and methodology, and – conversely – studies that employ advanced instruments and methodology are often difficult to implement on a large scale.

Given this tension and the current situation, the field of treatment evaluation at European level may best be served by a three-pronged approach:

- In line with the Pompidou Group's effort to establish a definitive treatment-demand protocol, modules may be developed to obtain core data not only on basic client characteristics, but also on basic programme, process and outcome characteristics.

- A number of key projects should be initiated at European level, aimed at further developing advanced instruments that lend themselves to standardised data collection in the areas of client, programme, process and outcome variables (the COST-A6 development of the European Addiction Severity Index (EuropASI – see Chapter 10 below) is a good example).

- Pilot studies should be conducted to test these advanced instruments in the context of innovative evaluation strategies. Such studies should involve selected European treatment centres.

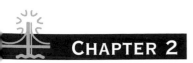

CHAPTER 2

TREATMENT-EVALUATION LITERATURE

Petra Paula Merino

A literature review undertaken by the EMCDDA's Demand-Reduction Department to identify relevant treatment-evaluation literature revealed three major trends. One concerned scientific investigation, another managerial and economic interest, and the third clinical practice.

Evidence of efficacy: scientific evaluation

Treatment interventions in the drugs field vary widely across, and even within, countries. Often, these interventions are selected more for political or administrative reasons than because of their actual effectiveness. In addition, concrete evidence of the benefits of targeting different approaches to different groups is lacking. In an attempt to redress this balance and to raise awareness of the effects of various treatment approaches, scientists have attempted to standardise the way information used in treatment-evaluation studies is collected and recorded. The two most commonly used techniques in evaluation research are retrospective, often naturalistic analyses, and prospective studies, either controlled clinical trials or randomised clinical trials. A third, less commonly used method is modelling.

Health-care and treatment approaches based on concrete evidence are becoming more widespread. Such evidence is particularly important for guiding health-care policy-makers, and information can be derived from overviews, structured reviews or meta-analyses of clinical trials. The statistical data thus collected can be analysed to give an overall picture of a particular intervention, allowing conclusions to be drawn that would not be possible if data from a single trial were analysed. In the field of drug abuse, the Cochrane collaboration – involving participants from all over the world and from different drug-related disciplines – is establishing a group to review the existing literature on substance abuse. In doing so, it will amass evidence from all the relevant randomised-controlled and clinical-controlled trials in the field.

From the scientific perspective, however, four major obstacles to treatment evaluation remain:

- the non-comparability of research findings;
- disagreement about what constitutes successful treatment outcome;
- the various measures used, specifically those related to drug use; and
- the general absence of control groups.

The non-comparability of research findings

One of the major methodological problems facing drug-treatment-evaluation literature is that research findings are often not comparable. In an attempt to combat this difficulty, much effort is being made to collect information systematically on what works in drug-abuse treatment.

The reasons for the non-comparability of research findings include:

- a failure to compare like with like, and resistance to comparing competing approaches;
- different client pools;
- differences in timescales between programmes;
- differing views of the goals of treatment;
- the lack of a common language across disciplines to describe client populations, treatment progress and results; and
- using research techniques of unknown validity and reliability which are often unique to the particular study.

What constitutes a successful treatment outcome?

Another major problem is reaching consensus on what constitutes a successful treatment outcome. The majority of the literature views a successful outcome as the achievement of total abstinence from drug use. As such, many studies use the rate of total abstinence as the primary – and sometimes sole – criterion for evaluating a treatment as 'successful'. Some other studies similarly report the frequency of substance use, while still others record the time span involved and rates of relapse. In addition to abstinence and substance use, the employment and socio-psychological condition of clients may also be explored.

Research into the effectiveness of different treatment approaches tends to point to the need for better patient–treatment matching and care systems. If the chosen indicators of effectiveness do not match the patients' own criteria, these patients may leave the care institutions prematurely (Arino *et al.*, 1988). In much of the treatment-evaluation literature, there is a clear awareness of the need to modify the criteria currently used to match clients to appropriate treatment and to take the individual patient's needs into greater consideration.

Measures of drug use

The existence of various methods of measuring drug use is another feature of the evaluation of treatment. All these methods have their limitations, and little is currently known about their impact on the interpretation of treatment outcome (Martin *et al.*, 1989). In addition, different measures of drug use may produce different results, making cross-study comparisons difficult (Wells *et al.*, 1988). Since those who abuse psychoactive drugs tend not to confine their use to one single drug, the resultant drug-dependent behaviour exhibited can be very complex.

The general absence of control groups

The tendency in the studies identified by the EMCDDA's literature review is to assert that the change measured is due solely to the treatment intervention itself. Factors identified include the inclination to apply outcome measures only to those individuals remaining in treatment while ignoring drop-outs, and the general absence of control groups for ethical reasons. The ethics of using control groups made up of those with severe drug problems to whom no assistance is given is highly problematic. The study of drug-abuse treatment has frequently been divorced from the study of the drug user, who is generally viewed first and foremost as a treatment client rather than as a drug user. Nevertheless, the user in treatment is, in certain respects, atypical. As a result, looking at drug users' needs solely from the point of view of treatment services and the approaches they provide means that a significant amount of information about the users themselves that could be of great value in improving drug-treatment interventions is not taken into account. To identify the users' real needs requires going beyond the service that is already being provided.

Programme management: cost-effectiveness and economic evaluation

In the past decade, major improvements have been made to the quality of programme planning and management in health-care services. These include assessing users' needs and evaluating costs and effectiveness in a systematic way to create clear policies on allocating the resources available. Evaluating treatment approaches is now seen as an integral part of programme management rather than as a purely scientific function, as was the tendency previously. Cost-effectiveness evaluations may be undertaken for one of two reasons – accountability or 'improving quality'. Substance-use services can be evaluated on many levels, including treatment activities and components, treatment services, treatment programmes and agencies, and treatment systems (WHO, 1997).

In terms of accountability, treatment programmes are evaluated to demonstrate their effectiveness to the funding sources. Accurate evaluations are required to allow programmes to be differentiated and to advise policy-makers on the quality of the different interventions. Programme-designers and managers face growing pressure to balance the costs of delivering a service with its results. Cost-effectiveness is thus often viewed as auditing, and not as process evaluation. In most countries, economic evaluation is intended to maximise health care using available, and often limited, resources. A genuine economic evaluation requires two key elements:

- it must compare inputs or cost and outputs or effects; and
- it must compare alternative treatments.

Clinical practice: treatment-progress evaluation

There is a clear division between actual clinical methods and experimental investigations (Miller *et al.*, 1995). The former has determined the standards for clinical practice, while the latter has generated the majority of the controlled studies found in the literature.

With growing pressure to remain within ever-tightening budgets and to justify their actions to funders and other external bodies, clinicians may be unable to provide the necessary data about their particular service, especially if they are not involved in the process of evaluation. Furthermore, these practitioners are unlikely to create their own evaluation programmes because they do not wish to see external control imposed on their decision-making and because many current evaluations lack real clinical value.

In Europe, valid and reliable instruments are being sought to assess treatment outcome across a broad range of drug-related problems and so enhance cross-study comparability. There are, however, different views of which instruments can serve clinical purposes or objective research purposes (Darke *et al.*, 1992). Instruments are also used for specific objectives in service delivery, including its economic and managerial aspects.

From the clinicians' point of view, the ideal evaluation instrument should:

- have clinical and research applications;
- be brief and easy to administer;
- be usable by both medical and non-medical staff;
- be understandable to clients;
- define admission;
- match clients to the appropriate level of care; and
- measure treatment progress.

Conclusions

The literature available on the evaluation of drug-abuse treatment derives mostly from scientific research. Yet it is still rare for this knowledge to be transferred adequately from the scientific level to that of current European practice. As a result, treatment strategies based on little scientific evidence are still often used.

A considerable amount of the information likely to be gathered in the course of clinical practice is lost because of the difficulties encountered by professionals in registering data systematically.

Treatment evaluation can also help to improve the delivery of treatment services, including their managerial and economic aspects, but these types of evaluations appear less frequently in the literature. The development of innovative reporting mechanisms on the Internet, based on current evaluation practices to improve service delivery, should increase the culture of evaluating the treatment of drug abuse.

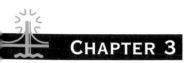

EVALUATING RESIDENTIAL
AND INSTITUTIONAL TREATMENT

Mats Fridell

Three basic concepts in evaluation research are often treated as if they were synonymous, despite the fact that they represent very different aspects of the process. These concepts are productivity, effectiveness and quality. The first two are fairly similar and can be assessed in economical and other objective terms. The concept of 'quality', on the other hand, involves a number of subjective and attitudinal factors, such as the needs and expectations of both the providers and 'consumers' of drug services. These concepts need to be defined if what it is that is being evaluated is to be understood.

Productivity describes the relationship between achievements and resources, while *effectiveness* is the relationship between effects and resources. The 'effectiveness' of a production unit can thus increase even if there is an overall decrease in existing resources ('rationalisation'). Cost-effectiveness can also increase when extra resources are made available, but only when the increase in effect is proportionally larger than the quantity of resources added. Finally, *quality* is the relationship between the actual level of service as experienced by its users and providers, and the expected level of quality (Dertell, 1989). In assessing quality, not only should the perspective of the treatment provider be taken into account, but also the subjective experiences of the treatment users – which are perhaps even more relevant. Scientific and pragmatic perspectives of 'quality' of service may well diverge markedly in such a situation.

To confuse the issue further, 'quality assurance' is another recent popular concept (Hansson *et al.*, 1993; Kelstrup *et al.*, 1993). Even if the concept itself lacks precision, it nevertheless indicates a need to consider objective issues alongside the assessment of clients' subjective experiences (Vuori, 1991). After assessing the quality of the ongoing treatment or its setting, the final stage is 'quality management'. This refers to the strategies used to implement and optimise quality goals (Fountain, 1992; Fridell, 1990). Systematic approaches, such as the 'client–treatment matching' described earlier, are promising – if not exhaustive – applications of quality management (McLellan *et al.*, 1983; MATCH Research Group, 1997).

Most evaluation studies focus on the effects of a defined intervention. 'Effect' and 'effectiveness' do not, however, refer to exactly the same domains. The latter concept might be used to indicate an increase in effect within the same treatment modality at a given point in time. In contrast, the former concept refers to the relative difference between two treatment methods or between a specific method and control groups which receive an alternative treatment or placebo. One of the main differences between the two concepts is that while methods to enhance effectiveness in one treatment setting may not easily be transposed to other settings, a randomised study of treatment effect can usually be compared to other treatment settings and groups. Such meta-analyses are measured in terms of 'efficacy' (Smith *et al.*, 1980; Crits-Christoph, 1992; Crits-Christoph and Siqueland, 1996).

However, in evaluating residential treatment, concepts such as 'effect' and 'efficacy' lose their precision, and it may be simpler to use the more modest term 'treatment outcome'.

Within an institution, such outcomes may be related to variations in the effectiveness of the intervention's implementation as well as to variations in client selection. Such a definition of 'outcome' may make it less easy to compare different treatment settings or modalities, but it remains a necessary ingredient for 'productivity control' and 'quality assurance' within the institution.

The problem of representativeness

In order to generalise research findings so that they can inform the whole treatment sector, patient-selection mechanisms need to be controlled. Samples entering different treatment modalities may differ substantially in outcome-dependent variables, such as psychopathology, gender or motivation.

Another problem facing evaluation studies is that many research concepts and techniques will be very imprecisely applied in the 'real world'. A specific therapeutic or pharmacological treatment may be applied very differently in the actual treatment setting than in a randomised control field trial, while issues familiar to researchers, such as 'consecutive samples', for example, are of little value if comparisons between experimental and control groups are lacking. Perhaps the only way around these difficulties is to regard the treatment modality itself as an *intermediate* rather than as an *independent* variable.

Randomised control design

As already outlined in Chapter 1, the method of choice in evaluating medical interventions is the so-called 'randomised control design'. This is easy to use in experimental animal research, because the 'learning curve' of the animals can be cut short by killing them so that skills learnt in one setting cannot be exported to another. Clearly, there could be problems if the same techniques were used in field settings on humans.

Alongside the ethical considerations touched on elsewhere in this monograph, another major methodological problem is that of internal consistency in data collection. The risk is that only some clients will be assessed on all the variables and across all the conditions, a situation that threatens the study's validity.

Furthermore, organisational variables must be included in controlled studies if any scientific explanation and interpretation of treatment outcome is to be made. A systematic application of this hypothesis on existing empirical research in residential settings was recently published by the author (Fridell, 1996a).

Finally, long-term follow-up is another dubious area when focusing on treatment effects, as changes over time in lifestyle and general socio-economic conditions must be expected to influence the individual's behaviour more than the specific treatment intervention made several years earlier.

These obvious problems, however, have done little to discourage randomised control trials (RCT). A recent Medline search from January 1998 included 647 studies defined as RCT on drug addiction only. Treatment studies on alcohol were not included. There were 90 studies of psychosocial treatment methods and ten RCT studies on institutional treatment as well as a large number of high-quality cohort studies (see, for example, Ravndal and Vaglum, 1992; Bale et al., 1980; Bell, 1985; McLellan et al., 1993; Woody et al., 1987). In addition to pharmacological studies on drug addiction, 247 RCTs were registered in Medline by January 1998. Reviews and meta-analyses of these psychosocial and pharmacological trials will be published by the Swedish Council on Technology Assessment in Health Care (SBU) in spring 1999.

The use of standardised instruments

The quality of any evaluation study – whether random controlled or otherwise – can be increased by consistently using a thorough common screen on all the clients, coupled with other standardised instruments that allow comparisons to be made between relevant client groups. This should also make it easier to compare the group against itself on a number of vital variables at follow-up.

It is important to pre-determine the validity and reliability of any assessment mechanism that was used in previous outcome studies. Anglo-American assessment instruments are most easily obtained at present, but any use of internationally accepted methods without good psychometric properties can only give a false basis for precision.

Although such instruments are plentiful in the alcohol field, they are not quite as common when it comes to drug use. Perhaps the most prevalent (and most regularly tested for validity and reliability) today is the Addiction Severity Index (ASI), which has been translated into a number of European languages. As Chapter 10 shows, a European version, EuropASI, has also been developed.

The ASI is used for individual assessment as well as group description, screening and follow-up (McLellan et al., 1980, 1985, 1992; Kosten et al., 1992). Long as well as short versions are available, and it has been adapted for various abusing groups, such as the homeless or young people (Friedman and Utada, 1989). ASI can be easily combined with other measures like the Symptom Check-List 90 (SCL-90 – Derogatis and Lipman, 1973; Derogatis, 1994) and the American Psychiatric Association's *Diagnostic and Statistical Manual of Mental Disorders* (DSM) diagnoses.

As personality disorders are diagnosed for 65–85% of clinical groups, and 30–60% have been found to have moderate-to-severe depressive and anxiety disorders, personality-assessment instruments must be included (Fridell, 1990, 1991, 1996b). The most frequently used diagnostic systems for personality disorders are the third edition, revised, and the fourth edition of the DSM (DSM-III-R and DSM-IV), facilitating international and national comparisons of patient groups. The diagnoses can be assessed either by clinical or by standardised interviews (Skodol *et al.*, 1988; Skre *et al.*, 1991).

As the DSM system is based entirely on a description of an individual's behaviour, clustered into sub-categories, it does not measure personality traits. A number of theory-based personality inventories and tests have therefore been developed to complement the formal DSM diagnoses. These inventories vary, however, as to their sensitivity in measuring change, their theoretical perspectives and their construct validity. Some are very stable over long periods of time, while others are more sensitive to change. Scales and tests should thus be selected on the basis of the primary research issue.

The most frequently used scale today is the Minnesota Multiphasic Personality Inventory (MMPI – Craig, 1979, 1980). Several hundred studies have employed MMPI data and a number of abbreviated scales exist, as well as some that have been specifically tailored to drug-related personality problems (Fridell, 1991).

Other scales that reflect severe personality disorders include Gunderson's Differential Diagnosis for Borderline and a Swedish implementation of Kernberg's tripartite model of psychological organisation, the Rating Ego Balance (Sandell, 1994). The latter has been used for epidemiological diagnostic purposes on large numbers of social-welfare clients with substance disorders in Stockholm (Bertling *et al.*, 1993; Sandell and Bertling, 1996). Still in Sweden, the Cesarec Marke Personality Scheme measures psychogenic need (Cesarec and Marke, 1968; Bech *et al.*, 1986; Hallstrom *et al.*, 1986; Holmlund, 1990). A short inventory measuring Basic Character Traits has also been developed over the last 15 years and is presently being standardised for large-scale use (Kline and Storey, 1977; Sandler and Hazari, 1960; Cesarec, 1980; Cesarec and Fridell, 1997). Another frequently used instrument is the Eysenck Personality Inventory (Eysenck, 1959; Eysenck and Eysenck, 1964), while the Karolinska Scale of Personality is also used, largely on alcoholic groups (Klinteberg *et al.*, 1986). Finally, the Psychopathy Checklist – Revised is, in this author's view, an underrated although internationally acclaimed psychiatric scale. It is of great value for studying drug dependence where anti-social behaviour can be easily confused with stable psycho-pathic traits, a factor which complicates the interpretation of test results and their application (Hare *et al.*, 1991; Klinteberg *et al.*, 1992).

Various promising scales also deal with the social network of drug misusers. In Sweden, the Australian-developed Individual Schedule for Social Integration has been widely applied (Henderson et al., 1980; Undén and Orth-Gomér, 1989; Orth-Gomér and Johnson, 1987).

Finally, returning to evaluating organisations and residential treatment, measuring the 'therapeutic climate in an organisation' has proved to be a meaningful and scientifically valid approach. The kind of measurements obtained involve staff as well as clients. The rationale is that organisational factors such as 'climate' and 'culture' reflect the selection of patients, staff competence, working relations and conflict levels. The most common instrument is the Ward Atmosphere Scale (Moos and Houts, 1968; Friis, 1986; Collins et al., 1985), which has been widely used in Scandinavian residential treatment studies.

In summary, for any form of evaluation, a number of different measurement instruments should be applied, for instance, self-assessment questionnaires, interview data and register data which should be used simultaneously. A research design of this kind is usually known as 'method triangulation' (Cook and Cambell, 1986).

Influencing outcome

Just as it involves a wide array of instruments and theories, evaluating drug treatment includes many design problems, complicating the comparability of treatments.

Spontaneous remission

One of the most influential myths that still survives today was launched by Charles Winnick in the early 1960s. He tracked substance misusers on New York State's narcotic registers, and those that were listed in the mid-1950s, but did not appear five years later, were classified as cases of 'spontaneous remission' (Winnick, 1962, 1964). Interestingly, an early repeat of this study could not support his very optimistic figures (Snow, 1973).

A number of prognostic studies on drug abuse exist, but one of the more qualified reviews reached very different conclusions from those of Winnick (Maddux and Desmond, 1980). This study found that the levels of possible spontaneous remission were very seldom greater than 20%. This author's own overview of existing data concludes that spontaneous remission is in the range of 10–15% (Fridell, 1991).

When evaluating the impact of 'spontaneous remission' on any treatment, the client base must be taken into account, as must the quality and quantity of an individual's social network. Schizophrenic drug misusers may have spontaneous remission rates of 0%, while maybe 95% of adolescents experimenting with drugs will spontaneously remit (Fridell, 1996b).

The drug that is being misused is another factor in evaluating 'spontaneous remission'. Prognostic studies of opiate users indicate a much lower level of abstinence at follow-up than is the case with other drugs. According to Haastrup and his colleagues, in the 1970s and 1980s early death was in fact the main factor contributing to the 'decrease' in opiate misuse at cohort follow-up (Haastrup and Jensen, 1988).

Attrition

Twenty years ago, the drop-out rate from treatment was extraordinarily high and outcome was often calculated for a mere 10–15% of the original patient cohort. However, it was also found that well-functioning institutions had lower drop-out rates than poorly functioning ones. Thus, by the, 1980s, some therapeutic communities were beginning to succeed in lowering drop-out considerably (Vaglum, 1979; Berglund et al., 1991). Today, it seems that some 30–40% of clients graduate from treatment, while studies also indicate a minimum length of treatment of 3–6 months before any substantial change takes place (DeLeon, 1991). The 'best' drop-out rates this author has come across are from a therapeutic community in New York, organised around the ideas of Daniel Casriel, with an annual drop-out rate of just 20% (Winnick, 1962).

One of the more substantial conclusions drawn from 30 years of research is that drug abusers recover as a function of time in treatment. This also seems to be the case for those dropping out of treatment (DeLeon, 1984; Condelli and Hubbard, 1994). To keep the individual in the treatment system, therefore, seems to be vital to the outcome. Of about 50 empirical studies supporting this conclusion, only one to date has presented an opposing view (McCusker et al., 1995). However, which variables predict drop-out is still unclear (Fridell, 1991). A recent multi-centre study comparing 'static' factors (such as gender, age and drug of misuse) with 'dynamic' factors (contact at admission interview, etc.) found that the best predictor of retention was the interviewer's rating of client motivation (Condelli and Hubbard, 1994). This was followed by whether the client spent most of the time with groups of people or preferred being alone. The third most important variable was external pressure to seek treatment.

So far, few studies have accounted for the influence of organisational variables on treatment outcome. But, as personality disorders are the dominant problem among drug-dependent patients, treatment structure and programme clarity remain factors of major importance (Fridell, 1990, 1996b; Ravndal, 1995).

Single or multiple criteria

The classic drug-treatment perspective is that the client must improve in more respects than just their use of drugs. There is considerable empirical support for such a position today. The most relevant – and pessimistic – application of multiple criteria is a model presented by the SWEDATE project, using cumulative criteria (Berglund et al., 1991). This found that a follow-up which only took into account abstinence from drugs had a general success rate of 50%. When alcohol use is added, this level decreases to 40%. If successively more and more criteria are included, the rehabilitation figures plummet and, finally, only some 10–14% will be completely rehabilitated and free from psychological suffering.

It is important to note, however, that several misconceptions are built into such a critical appraisal. The first is that medical and psychological treatment never expect a person to be completely cured. The second, and perhaps more important, issue is that such a criterion as psychological well-being is inappropriate, as only 40% of heavy drug misusers at a recent five-year follow-up fulfilled this criterion, regardless of whether they were abstinent at this point or not (Fridell *et al.*, 1996). On the positive side, several recent reviews of the treatment of heavy drug use have concluded that success rates in treating substance disorders are as high or higher than in many other chronic ailments (O'Brien and McLellan, 1996; O'Brien, 1996; Crits-Cristoph and Siqueland, 1996).

Short- or long-term follow-up

A common ideal is to discuss outcome in terms of one- or two-year follow-ups. Very often shorter-term perspectives, such as goal attainment at discharge from acute or short-term rehabilitating services, are overlooked. This creates problems when trying to compare levels of goal attainment in, for example, psychiatric departments and therapeutic communities. Differences in goals and focus must therefore be taken into consideration.

On the other hand, patients admitted to a psychiatric ward can be expected to have more severe as well as longer-term problems. The need to train staff to maintain good-quality care for these patients is clearly vital if future and long-term treatment efforts are to be motivated. Quality of treatment (and sometimes its lack) is probably as important in the short term as it is in the long term, even though the foci of treatment vary.

Simple goal-attainment procedures can therefore be highly relevant when measuring short-term interventions (Kiresuk and Sherman, 1968; Kiresuk, 1973). Goal attainment is, in its own right, a rather sensitive measure of organisational stability, and it has been successfully used to increase staff participation in the treatment setting (Fridell, 1990). It is important to note that an unmotivated patient can be positively motivated by an empathetic staff member and, likewise, that a motivated patient can lose motivation because of indifferent 'care'.

The quality of daily care thus needs to be high, regardless of the fact that it might not increase long-term outcome as far as is known today. An illustration of this is a randomised control study from Finland which compared treatment in a therapeutic community with the ambulatory treatment of heavy problem drinkers (Keso and Salaspuro, 1990). All the patients were included in the study, and one-year follow-up found a somewhat larger improvement for those in residential treatment. These patients generally reported a higher level of satisfaction with treatment, which was also reflected in a more positive evaluation of institutional climate as measured by the Ward Atmosphere Scale. The differences in complete abstinence and controlled drinking between the two groups, however, were not significant.

This illustrates the difference between the satisfaction of quality experienced in a defined setting and the issue of treatment outcome. The study does not, however, answer the question of which treatment is best. To do so, a representative sample of therapeutic communities must be compared to a representative sample of ambulatory care facilities.

Conclusions

Despite the vast amount of treatment-evaluation literature, a number of misconceptions still exist. The first is that treatment strategies in general are ineffective and that treatment yields only modest levels of success. However, empirical research demonstrates that treatment can be very effective, and several recent reviews show a considerable success rate using psychosocial and therapeutic modalities (Crits-Christoph and Siqueland, 1996). The problem is more one of *intra*-modality variation (between, for example, US and UK therapeutic-community models) rather than one of *inter*-modality variation (for example, between therapeutic communities and psychiatric in-patient units).

Despite this evidence, the problems of evaluation still cause heated debate and engender a number of conflicting views. One of these is the reference to what should be regarded as a basic 'non-treatment level', such as the issue of high spontaneous remission. Another is that evaluation itself has demonstrated that drug misusers are a more heterogeneous group than was previously believed. Questions about proper comparison groups, self-selection, spontaneous remission and the type and degree of psychiatric disorder have consequently become more and more pertinent, and more vital to interpreting outcome.

Over the last decade, much attention has been paid to client–treatment matching factors, such as psychiatric disorders, gender or other specific subgroup issues, since these areas might indicate the need for a specific intervention, increasing the probability of a successful outcome. The need for a diverse continuum of criteria for treatment evaluation is therefore necessary, especially where the otherwise obvious goal of abstinence might be secondary to reducing risky behaviour or stabilising psychiatric symptoms.

This chapter has examined some of the most central issues in evaluating residential treatment. Different and complementary research approaches must also be considered, whether the basic aim is to study effects, outcome or quality assurance. No single research design provides answers to all these diverse fields, and many – if not most – of the problems related to institutional treatment might be better approached by models other than the standard procedures of randomised control studies.

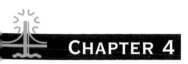

CHAPTER 4

METHODOLOGICAL ASPECTS
OF TREATMENT EVALUATION

Fabio Mariani

In any thorough evaluation of drug treatment, it is crucial to define the characteristics of those people undergoing the treatment. It is commonly assumed, however, that 'abuse' and 'dependence' – perhaps the most fundamental characteristics of anyone being treated for drug problems – are almost impossible to define, observe, measure or differentiate. This assumption is erroneous, as much of the research over the last 40 years has demonstrated.

That said, it can be difficult to distinguish between 'abuse' and 'dependence' in an individual, as so much hinges on the personality of the user and the relationship between drug use, dependence and socio-cultural aspects. Physiological and environmental factors, together with drug careers ('drug, set, setting'), are the most familiar of the many confounding factors that can influence the evaluation of treatment effects.

In the American Psychiatric Association's *Diagnostic and Statistical Manual of Mental Disorders* (DSM), the concept of a 'psychoactive substance dependence disorder' is defined as undesirable behaviour associated with regular drug use, rather than as an acute or chronic drug reaction. The *Manual's* account of substance dependence is simply a codification of common sense. People who display a number of the following symptoms are said to be 'dependent' on a drug:

- repeatedly taking more than intended or for longer than intended;
- knowing they are using too much, but being unable to stop;
- spending much of their time either obtaining the drug, intoxicated or recovering from the drug's effects;
- being unable to fulfil social, familial and work obligations because of intoxication;
- giving up most other activities in order to use drugs;
- continuing to take the drug although they know it is damaging their health, working capacity or family life;
- developing tolerance, making it necessary to raise the dose to preserve the original effect;
- withdrawal symptoms; and
- constant use of the drug to relieve or avoid withdrawal symptoms.

Comparative evaluation and confounding factors

The 'perfect treatment' is an unattainable holy grail. Undesired and unplanned short- and long-term collateral effects will always affect a treatment for some people in some particular application or circumstance. In such cases, it is vital to evaluate all possible outcomes, whether positive or negative, and not just those that are the object of study. Generally speaking, it is also inadvisable to examine the efficacy of one treatment to the exclusion of all others as there are many treatment modalities, each with their own measures of effectiveness and efficiency.

Effectiveness evaluation must therefore be comparative, as it is necessary to demonstrate how – and to what extent – one particular treatment is 'better' than another. If no other treatments are available, the treatment being evaluated should be compared with the natural evolution of the situation, either in the absence of therapy or in the presence of a placebo.

The advantage of a comparison with a placebo 'treatment' rather than with natural evolution is that it aims to counter the psychological effect of treatment. The main hurdle to this type of comparative study is the problem of implementing the study protocol effectively in a 'double-blind' procedure in which neither those submitted to the placebo nor those 'treating' them know that they are in this situation.

A further important point is the near impossibility of finding treatments or placebos that can be adequately compared. Consequently, the judgement of effectiveness will tend to be established as a probability of success, estimated by the ratio between the number of cases with favourable outcomes and the total number admitted to treatment. For this reason, it is important to know if the distribution of positive outcomes in the treated group is related solely to the treatment modality or whether it is related to other factors or causal effects.

Finally, two other aspects which could influence the choice of treatment need to be considered. The first factor is whether a particular treatment is the 'best fit' for the client group. If so, proof of its efficacy should be available for subjects with similar characteristics. The second factor – and one without which no treatment evaluation can be effectively performed – is the acceptability of the treatment to the client.

Randomised control trials

As already stated, the best way to evaluate an untried treatment is to organise the study with two experimental subject groups, the first being submitted to the treatment, and the second ('the control group') to a placebo or already-evaluated treatment. This could include prevention programmes, rehabilitation, in-patient and outpatient interventions, and true placebos.

For the evaluation to have any scientific validity, subjects must be assigned randomly to the two experimental groups, although the full 'pool' of subjects should be as similar as possible and certain factors should be identified as 'matching' variables to avoid any confounding factors or an uneven weighting between the two groups. The best way to do this is to work with the most specific group of subjects as is practicable. Similar age ranges, gender distribution, substance-use history, family situation, socio-economic and psychological characteristics should all be considered, so that the final assignment to either group can be a true picture of the target client population.

The more time and effort that is spent characterising, defining and limiting the target population the more specific that population becomes and the easier it is to limit the number of variables under consideration. On the other hand, the wider the group, the more difficult it is to define objective criteria to describe their characteristics and measure treatment outcomes. One method that is frequently employed to define the groups is to stratify the sample in terms of prognostic factors, during both enrolment and data analysis.

Stratification during enrolment allows for an increase in statistical accuracy as the main exclusion of confounding factors takes place at the outset, allowing clinical outcome to be closely related to the prognostic factor. Stratification during data analysis, however, risks limiting the evaluation to extremely small numbers of subjects. For example, if at this stage three main strata were defined (gender, age and clinical factors) which all had a number of internal strata (male/female; <18 years, 18–24, >25 years; opiate use, polydrug use) then by the end of the process there would be 3 x 2 x 2 strata for each experimental group, in other words, 24 strata in total. The likelihood of finding many subjects in the same strata would therefore be extremely low.

Defining the inclusion criteria

Clearly, any evaluation must begin by defining precise criteria for including its subjects in the study. Client characteristics and methodologies for data collection should also be defined at this stage. Moreover, all subjects presenting specific contra-indications for any of the treatments under examination should be excluded. For example, seropositivity and the possible development of AIDS cannot be ignored when providing certain treatments, especially placebo 'treatment'.

If the aim of the study is simply to select a treatment that is more effective than another, inclusion criteria can be less strict than when the aim is to compare and elucidate different modalities of action within different treatments. In any case, both the diagnosis and the severity of the pathology should be defined for each subject to allow for analysis according to accuracy and repeatability.

Defining the therapeutic protocol

One of the most important aspects of research is the possibility of repeating a study in various contexts. In the context of treatment evaluation, this requires a detailed definition of therapeutic protocols for different treatments. In the case of drug dependence, the physiological and social aspects of clinical, biological, pharmacological and compliance issues also need to be considered.

Defining the major outcomes

Drug-free behaviour is clearly the ultimate desirable outcome when considering any treatment evaluation. But to characterise such behaviour better, a number of secondary outcomes on the road to abstinence must be defined.

In general, a certain variability exists between professions when formulating any diagnosis, defining prognostic factors or describing outcomes. For an effective evaluation, all these possible criteria must not only be clearly defined, but also capable of objective measurement. Observations made by professionals should therefore be accurate (in other words, close to the phenomenon being observed) and easy to repeat (observations of different professionals concerning the same issue and of the same professional at different times should elicit the same results). All the variables under consideration should be examined using standard criteria and modalities, and any new criterion should also take account of accuracy and repeatability.

In any multi-site study, and often in longitudinal studies too, quality control is vital. If the outcomes under evaluation can be subject to differing professional theoretical conceptions, it is important to guarantee that data collection is performed by researchers with no stake in the outcome. In other words, they have to be part of the 'double-blind' aspect of the study, having no past knowledge of the treatment under evaluation.

Confounding factors

One of the major sources of distortion during any evaluation study is the unforeseen impact of additional diagnostic and therapeutic factors not considered by the original protocol. This kind of distortion is of particular concern in the drug field, as even small, apparently unrelated variations in a subject's micro or macro environment (such as family tension) can have far-reaching effects.

Effect of drop-out on data analysis

Knowing what has happened to those who have dropped out of treatment is just as important as knowing about those who have remained in the study. Clearly, if they have left it may be impossible to follow them up, but it is usual to 'cancel them out' against individuals who complete treatment. For example, a positive outcome should be applied if the drop-outs belonged to the group showing overall negative reactions, and a negative outcome should be applied if they belonged to the group with more positive reactions.

Clinical and statistical significance

Clinical significance refers to the importance placed by researchers on the differences in clinical developments between the two groups under comparison – for instance, in relation to the incidence of relapse, mortality or seroconversion.

Statistical significance, on the other hand, only indicates that the observed difference is probably related to the treatment, without implying any judgement as to the clinical value of the variation.

Other forms of evaluation study

A number of other experimental, as well as observational, studies can be used in treatment evaluation when randomised control trials are seen to be impossible or inappropriate.

As already stated, in experimental studies the researcher defines the inclusion criteria for making up groups, as well as criteria for selecting treatment. In observational studies, on the other hand, the effects of treatment are simply analysed without any specific research design.

Observational studies can be useful when a body of experimental evidence already exists and the effectiveness of the routine application of a treatment needs to be assessed. But, whatever the case, when choosing a particular study design it should always be remembered that whenever the scientific basis for a treatment being better than another is low, greater methodological accuracy is needed.

Non-randomised control studies

This form of experimental design is similar to that already described, the only difference being that inclusion in a particular group and enrolment in treatment are not random.

In this case, researchers explicitly assign subjects to the different treatments. It is therefore necessary to conform to strict inclusion/exclusion criteria in order to make the groups as similar as possible regarding known prognostic characteristics and to allow comparability between them.

Pre- and post-test studies

Other studies examine subjects before and after treatment, measuring any improvement. The issue of whether a possible outcome can be ascribed to the treatment is of great significance here, however, as confounding factors are more likely to occur when 'time' is taken into account.

Retrospective studies

This evaluation model examines data on groups of subjects submitted to different past treatments. The main advantage is that a large number of subjects can be considered over a greater timescale and geographical spread.

The main disadvantage, however, is that, as the events have already taken place, a number of essential data elements can be missing. These may include:

- the standardisation of therapeutic protocols;
- the definition of inclusion criteria;
- the accuracy and completeness of individual data related to the prognosis;
- the standardisation of outcome measures;
- the evaluation of all subjects, including drop-outs; and
- the effects of unforeseen confounding factors.

Case-control studies

The most frequent application of case-control studies is when a causal relationship between etiological and protective factors is being examined. Usually the 'cases' are subjects displaying the factor being examined, while the 'controls' are subjects without this condition.

Case studies

Finally, studies can be carried out with no control, examining only those subjects admitted to the treatment under evaluation. As such a study cannot compare the treatment to any other, its main application is to develop new hypotheses about treatment and outcomes.

Conclusions

The randomised control trial seems to be the best choice for assessing drug treatment, both because of its methodological aspects and because of the reliability of its results.

Nevertheless, even control studies face a number of operational difficulties:

- the difficulty inherent in defining and standardising objective methods which can be applied across the different professions involved for describing and assessing client characteristics;
- the impossibility of controlling factors not covered by the protocol, but which can still modify the subject's condition and its evolution over time; and
- the low level of statistical and epidemiological competence among professionals working in the field.

Any future improvement in the quality of drug treatment in Europe must, therefore, rest on further evaluation research. Improving epidemiological and statistical competence among drug professionals can also be seen as a positive step. The European Monitoring Centre for Drugs and Drug Addiction can play a major role in facilitating study design and the statistical analysis of epidemiological data, both of which are essential for the future of effective treatment.

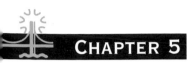

CHAPTER 5

APPLYING ECONOMIC EVALUATION
IN THE SUBSTANCE-MISUSE FIELD

Evi Hatziandreou

The constant battle between competing needs for society's scarce health-care and social resources is clear for all to see. These resources are not, however, only financial: people, facilities, equipment, time and even knowledge are all finite, and alternative uses for them can be found both within and without the health-care sector. This situation dictates that choices need to be made as to how best to use resources.

In economics, this is the notion of 'opportunity cost' – the value of the best alternative which is foregone because the resources available were used for other purposes. In other words, the real cost of any programme is not simply its budget, but also the health and social outcomes that have not been achieved by some other programme because resources have been devoted to another project. Society's goal is to maximise the total benefits (health, social, etc.) of these finite resources. Efficiency is achieved when a given amount of available resources produces as much 'effectiveness' or benefit as possible or, alternatively, when a specified goal is achieved at the lowest cost. The desire for efficiency is the driving force behind economic evaluation. This scientific discipline is of the utmost relevance to health and social decision-making at all levels, as it provides the necessary economic and social data for informed decisions to be made. In recent years, the importance of economic evaluation has been strengthened by the competitive marketplace, the demand for accountability, the desire to assess the return on investments and the need to allocate resources as wisely as possible.

Economic evaluation identifies, measures, values and compares the costs and consequences of alternative uses of finite resources (Drummond *et al.*, 1987). It examines in an organised, systematic and explicit way all the factors involved in a decision to commit resources to one form of action rather than another. In this way, it deals explicitly with the issue of 'choice'. Therefore, if treatment is to achieve its potential, so too must economic evaluation. This chapter introduces the key concepts involved and illustrates the uses to which economic evaluation can – and must – be put.

Definitions

According to Drummond *et al.* (1987), two fundamental and interdependent questions face decision-makers and funders:

- Is it worthwhile allocating scarce resources to a health procedure, service, programme or intervention?
- Could the resources thus allocated be spent more productively?

Economic evaluation can help to answer these questions. It is a structured, systematic, comprehensive and explicit process which establishes the context of the problem, lays out the alternatives, predicts the consequences of each alternative, values the expected outcomes and calculates their total costs and benefits.

In the health sector, this is accomplished by determining the total value of a specific programme. The value of improved health is reflected in a number of ways. Better health reduces the need for health care and conserves resources. It increases productivity by lowering absenteeism and improving worker output. It also has the inherent value of influencing the length and quality of an individual's life. But for the decision-maker, its main value is its ability to improve the consistency and quality of decision-making.

Rationale for economic evaluation

Drummond *et al.* (1987)'s two general questions can form the basis for the issues covered by economic evaluation:

- can this intervention work – a question of 'efficacy';
- does this intervention work – a question of 'effectiveness'; and
- does this intervention reach those who need it – a question of 'availability'.

As the other chapters in this monograph show, the distinction between 'efficacy' and 'effectiveness' is key to evaluation. The former assesses the likelihood of the benefit to individuals in a defined population as a result of a specific intervention applied to a given health or social problem under ideal conditions. The latter refers to the expected outcomes under realistic conditions.

The availability of – and access to – an intervention is also a matter for economic evaluation (Plotnick, 1994). It is important to consider how 'costs' and 'benefits' (or social gains and losses) are distributed among the different sections of society, just as it is important to understand from whose perspective the costs and benefits are examined. If this societal view is adopted, all the significant costs and benefits that flow from the intervention are taken into account, regardless of who is experiencing them.

Costs and health benefits

Costs are defined as the economic resources used to provide a service. There are three categories of cost:

- *direct costs*, which measure the value of resources directly consumed. These costs can be health- and/or non-health-related;
- *indirect costs*, which reflect the value of lost or reduced productivity due to premature mortality or morbidity; and

- *intangible costs*, the hardest to measure, related to the suffering, stress and isolation of those in ill health (in this case, drug dependence).

The major components of substance misuse costs are (French *et al.*, 1991; Plotnick, 1994):

- health-care costs;
- criminal-justice costs;
- social-service costs; and
- other hidden costs, such as those resulting from aversive behaviour (the installation of security systems, for example) and personal and psychological costs.

Health benefits may take many forms, for example: prolonged life; improved functioning and activity; relief from pain and anxiety; greater capacity to work and earn; reduced medical-care expenses; and enhanced quality of life.

Types of economic evaluation

Economic evaluation encompasses different analytical approaches with some common methodological features (Drummond *et al.*, 1987): those that only measure costs; and those that measure both costs and health benefits. A third category measures health-related quality of life but is not discussed here.

Cost-only approaches

Cost of Illness (COI) studies are descriptive and aim to enumerate all the costs related to a specific disease or condition (whether asthma, cardiovascular disease, substance misuse, etc.) in the population in question. They therefore estimate the total economic burden on society of a condition, as opposed to the costs of a specific intervention. No comparison of alternative interventions Is involved. COI studies follow either a prevalence-based or incidence-based approach: the former estimates costs for a base year; the latter estimates lifetime costs associated with the condition.

Cost Minimisation Analysis (CMA) is used when the interventions being evaluated produce similar outcomes, sharing the same effectiveness. The least costly alternative is then identified by comparing the total costs of each. This is the simplest form of socio-economic analysis (Luce and Elixhauser, 1990), but it is important for this equivalence to be rigorously documented if a CMA is to be justified.

Cost–benefit approaches

A number of methodologies allow interventions which have differential outcomes to be compared. These methodologies differ, essentially, in the manner in which the benefits are measured. Obviously, for such studies to work, the expected differential benefits from alternative uses of available resources need to be known.

Cost–Benefit Analysis (CBA) enumerates and compares the costs and benefits of a particular intervention. Its distinguishing feature is that both costs and benefits are measured in *monetary* terms. This approach attempts to determine whether an intervention's expenditure is greater or lower than its expected benefits, also measured financially. The cost–benefit ratio, which calculates benefit minus cost, is then used to evaluate the intervention – if the ratio is positive, then society is better off devoting resources to that particular intervention.

In contrast, Cost-Effectiveness Analysis (CEA) does not convert health and social outcomes into monetary units. This is particularly appropriate when monetary values for the principal benefits are not quantifiable or are controversial. In contrast, CEA quantifies these benefits in the most appropriate health or physical units, such as days of morbidity averted, the number of cases prevented or years of life saved. Treatment-related benefits could include the number of abstinent incidents over time or a specific reduction in drug use or crime. At the end of this process, a cost-effectiveness ratio is calculated, being the cost per specified health-effectiveness unit. CEA can therefore depict the trade-offs involved when choosing between different interventions or variations of an intervention, although only interventions with outcomes measured in equivalent units can be compared (Gold *et al.*, 1996).

Similarly, Cost-Utility Analysis (CUA) compares two or more interventions, measuring costs in monetary terms, but also considering benefits in terms of quality or utility (Luce and Elixhauser, 1990). CUA does not simply enumerate these benefits as 'years of life saved', but uses a broader analytical framework. Unlike CEA, only one outcome measure, the 'quality-adjusted life years' (QALYs), allows interventions with non-equivalent outcome units to be compared.

Economic evaluation in drug treatment

Despite the fact that resources have traditionally been scarce, and although economic evaluation is an irreplaceable tool when seeking to maximise collective benefits, it has rarely been applied systematically to the drug-treatment field. There are a number of notable exceptions, however.

Cost of Illness

Over the past 20 years, numerous studies have assessed the economic costs of drug misuse. According to various researchers (French *et al.*, 1991; President's Commission on Model State Drug Laws, 1993), these studies have significantly underestimated the true burden on society by failing to consider tangible expenses that affect the drug user, the environment and society at large. These sums may include falling property values in drug-using communities, the real and opportunity costs of drug-education programmes and the financial effects of complications related to secondary disease. Similarly, because of the difficulty and controversy surrounding the methods used to measure intangible costs, these have rarely been included.

A distinct feature of the costs of drug misuse (as opposed to those of alcohol misuse and mental illness) is the high proportion, up to 74% in some studies, of crime-related expenses (Rice *et al.*, 1991). This is strong evidence that society, and not the individual, bears the burden of the economic consequences of drug misuse. It is also worthwhile noting the observation of researchers at Rutgers University (President's Commission on Model State Drug Laws, 1993) that, while up to 41% of the total cost of illness is borne directly by treatment and treatment-support services in the mental-health field, less than 5% of drug-misuse expenditure is borne by addiction treatment.

COI studies and methodologies *have* improved (see French and colleagues, 1996). This provides a comprehensive conceptual framework to help researchers more accurately estimate the social costs of drug misuse. The process is made more uniform by capturing tangible and intangible costs that were previously left out.

The first step of this framework calls for categorising the adverse health and non-health consequences of drug misuse into one of three classes: physical-health problems; mental-health problems; and social problems. The second step identifies and classifies the associated costs by their bearer. Finally, methods to estimate each of the social-cost components need to be selected and developed.

Cost–Benefit and Cost-Effectiveness Analysis

COI studies can estimate the aggregate monetary burden to society of the health and social effects of drug misuse. Inherently, however, they do not contain information that decision-makers can use to assist them in resource allocation. This is the domain of CBA and CEA.

Relatively few CBA and CEA studies have been conducted in the drug-treatment field. In a critical assessment of the existing literature, Apsler (1991) claims that there is no single and straightforward answer to the question: 'Are today's drug-treatment programmes cost-effective?' According to Cartwright and Kaple (1991), not only are some treatment programmes of 'questionable' cost-effectiveness, some are even 'cost-ineffective'. Underlying this lack of clarity is perhaps a lack of rigour in research design and implementation.

Recent methodological improvements do, however, parallel those in COI studies. A particularly interesting and relevant example is the work carried out, again, by French and colleagues (1996). These researchers developed a simple methodology to estimate the health-related costs of drug misuse based on a rigorous theoretical foundation. They used an integrated approach combining medicine, epidemiology, economics and psychology, aimed at a target group of policy analysts, evaluators and researchers.

The technique developed uses QALYs to estimate the value of avoiding drug-related morbidity and mortality. The methodology is then tested by estimating the value of avoiding sexually transmitted diseases, hypertension, bacterial pneumonia and tuberculosis in a 32-year-old white American male. It is also important to mention Hser and Anglin's recommendation to use more sophisticated techniques, such as time-series analysis and advanced modelling, when assessing treatment impact (Hser and Anglin, 1991).

Overall, despite the lack of rigorous CBA or CEA studies, those available demonstrate that the benefits of treatment seem to be at least as great as the respective costs. Clearly, however, this evidence needs to be strengthened by further appropriately designed and conducted economic evaluations.

Methodological challenges

Economic evaluation is not an easy area for researchers. A plethora of obstacles and hurdles need to be overcome, especially as evidence of 'effectiveness' is more difficult to measure than 'cost'. Assigning an observed effect to treatment, the bias inherent in selection and self-selection, and the relative weakness of the evidence (contrasting, for example, with the role of drug-use careers) all pose formidable challenges. Apsler (1991) summarises these challenges as follows:

* conceptual problems;
* disagreement about treatment goals;
* disagreement about outcomes;
* duration of treatment;
* existing variability among different interventions;
* high drop-out rates; and
* an over-reliance on self-reports.

More 'manageable' difficulties include multidimensional and time-related consequences, as well as the problems associated with assigning monetary value to costs or benefits. Finally, the relevance of any results to untreated populations remains a dilemma that cannot be easily ignored.

To address these challenges, Apsler (1991) notes the importance of developing some form of standard methodology or guidelines. This could include establishing a working definition of treatment goals and deriving appropriate outcome measures from them. He also recommends developing a comprehensive set of objective measures for assessing outcomes.

Complementary activities have also been proposed to catalyse integrating economic evaluation into programme evaluation. These include educating decision-makers about economic evaluation, its purpose, nature, strengths and limitations. Furthermore, early exposure to the principles of economic evaluation should be encouraged for social scientists.

Ultimately, the burden of evidence is growing heavier. Policy-making now requires information and a sound understanding not only of the nature and magnitude of the real consequences of drug misuse, but also of the cost and effectiveness of alternative interventions, so as better to allocate resources. Economic evaluation can provide this and, in so doing, can make the decision process more explicit and transparent. But, if it is to do so, more sophisticated techniques and approaches urgently need to be developed.

TREATMENT EVALUATION IN PRACTICE

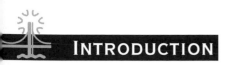

PART II

INTRODUCTION

*H*einrich Küfner begins this section by outlining how the principles of treatment evaluation can be applied in practice. In particular, he explores the barriers to the effective use of evaluation findings in the clinical setting, a situation that leaves the question 'what works?' unanswered. Küfner's suggestions for making evaluation relevant to the practitioner include setting research standards and classifying research designs. He also recommends systems theory as a way of rooting evaluation in the practitioner's experience of working with drug users.*

Umberto Nizzoli then illustrates how evaluation can be applied on the ground. Drawing on his experience developing an information system in the Emilia-Romagna region of Italy, he underlines the obstacles to strategic development, among them the lack of shared evaluation goals, opposition to the concept of evaluation, and never-ending discussions about the usefulness or otherwise of evaluating particular projects. Nizzoli goes on to describe how Emilia-Romagna developed its own evaluation instrument, TedEval, and how similar systems are being developed throughout Europe via inter- and intra-sectoral communication.

In the final chapter of this section, Michael Gossop and the National Treatment Outcome Research Study (NTORS) team detail how a treatment-evaluation system was set up in the UK, and describe the Maudsley Addiction Profile, an evaluation instrument developed specifically for NTORS. The Study now plays an important role in developing and guiding British drug-treatment policy responses. Its initial findings have provided the evidence that treating drug problems can reduce harm both to individuals and to society as a whole. These findings have also been used by the UK Department of Health to formulate guidance for treatment purchasers.

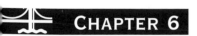

USING EVALUATION RESULTS
IN TREATING DRUG ADDICTION

Heinrich Küfner

The influence of evaluation research on treating drug addiction seems to be very limited. Whether, given the current state of evaluation research, it is desirable that research findings should have a stronger influence on the field or not requires more detailed consideration. There are many good reasons, on both the research and clinical sides, why the influence is not very great.

Problems and limitations of evaluation research

External validity

Outcome research often has a low external validity, meaning that any generalisation of results to other patient samples and treatment settings should be undertaken very cautiously. Patient samples should be representative for the population being assessed and statements about influence variables restricted to categories of those variables assessed in the studies. Figure 1 demonstrates the problem of assessing influence variables with insufficient variations.

Studies	Abstinence rank correlation (n studies)	Improved rank correlation (n studies)
All studies	0.35 (38)	0.14 (40)
Germany	0.50 (10)	0.33 (10)
Other countries	0.12 (28)	0.03 (30)

Figure 1: Treatment length and outcome in residential treatment

Source: Süß (1995)

In alcoholism research, Anglo-Saxon researchers have found no relationship between length of treatment and outcome (Miller *et al.*, 1995). A meta-analytic study including investigations about alcoholism treatment in Germany (Süß, 1995) demonstrated a low, but significant association between treatment length and positive outcome (r = 0.35). In German outcome studies, with their much longer treatment length, there was a substantial association of outcome with treatment length with a rank correlation coefficient of r = 0.52.

But excluding these German studies, Anglo-Saxon research found no significant relationship between the two as only treatments of less than 4–6 months' duration were studied. Thus, treatment length as a variable was not represented in the full range of clinically relevant variations. Significant relationships between outcome and treatment length cannot be proved purely by short-term treatment. Therefore, generalisation of these studies is restricted.

As for patient samples, the scientific ideal is that of a randomised control study. But, as has already been argued in previous chapters, such studies are not necessarily without bias – only patients who are willing to undergo any of the treatments on offer can be enrolled in the sample. In reality, substantial groups of patients are not willing to participate in the treatment alternatives being provided.

Internal validity

Another major problem with evaluation is that the results of outcome research are seldom clear, allowing instead for multiple interpretations. As a result, not only external but also internal validity may be insufficient. For example, there may be several competing causal explanations and interpretations for the results of an evaluation. In statistical terms, a low rate of explained variance of an outcome variable indicates the likelihood of many unknown influences. Furthermore, if the results are not conclusive it is hardly reasonable to draw far-reaching conclusions.

Discrepancies in results

Different studies into the same issue often do not produce similar results. It is thus unwise to rely on a single study. In the case of such discrepancies, the task facing researchers is to explain and accept the differences.

One option is to carry out meta-analyses as a quantitative method of summarising evaluation results. Although there may not always be a sufficient number of studies for meta-analyses, if several investigations concerning a particular variable do exist, meta-analysis is the best quantitative way to summarise the evaluation results (Durlake and Lipsey, 1991; Cartwright and Kaple, 1991). While meta-analysis does have several drawbacks, such as merging the results of studies carried out under different conditions, it can give more valid results than narrative reviews.

One condition for such an analysis is the existence of enough studies with corresponding outcome criteria. This may, however, prove problematic in the field of drug addiction. To date, as far as this author is aware, no meta-analytic study has been published into catamnestic treatment outcome in illegal drug addiction, although two reviews are in progress (one in the framework of the IPTRP project, co-ordinated by Kaplan and colleagues, and one by Prendergast, Podus and Chang, 1998). Several questions remain open about the methods of meta-analysis, but overall this approach would improve the present status of outcome research.

Insufficient differentiated outcome

In most cases, outcome research relates to global outcome criteria, for example to the categories 'improved' or 'unimproved' in relation to drug consumption and other such factors. Outcome is seldom related in a multivariate way to client or treatment characteristics and to external circumstances applying multivariate statistical tools.

On the other hand, the clinical tasks of diagnosis and treatment are tailored to a large extent to the patient's individual situation with its many influencing and confounding factors. These create many questions that cannot be answered by global outcome studies. To bridge the gap between clinical tasks and the scientific approach of evaluation is thus a continuous problem.

Divergent aims and interests

Evaluation research is often fragmented. Clinicians, for example, are more interested in the effect of individual treatment components – so that they can be added to or removed from existing treatment programmes – than in the total treatment package. To plan such studies over a longer time period, however, requires close co-operation between researchers and clinicians. Evaluation has to be applied as part of a clear strategy, for example, to improve a single treatment system or to improve a treatment system in a specific region or country. Despite the different political interests in evaluation results, the scientific criteria of reproducibility and objectivity have to be fulfilled.

Feedback to practitioners

A final issue is that there is all too often a long delay between data analysis and feedback to the clinicians, which can invalidate the research. If data are to be relevant for clinical decisions, for example a patient profile on the European Addiction Severity Index (EuropASI), they have to be fed back quickly. While this is never easy in the research field, the hardware and software are now available to facilitate this task.

Improving evaluation research

Besides these difficulties and limitations, it should be emphasised that there is no alternative to evaluation. There are, however, many opportunities for improving the situation.

First and foremost, it is essential to set research standards or to suggest solutions for methodological problems in treatment evaluation. Some ideas have already been proposed, for example in the National Institute on Drug Abuse Monograph series (Cázares and Beatty, 1994; Kolbey and Asghar, 1992) or by the German Association of Addiction Research and Treatment (Deutsche Gesellschaft für Suchtforschung und Suchttherapie e.V., 1994), but as far as this author knows, no European standards are yet available for illegal drugs.

Evaluation standards have only been actively developed in the prevention field (EMCDDA, 1998b), but there are clearly areas where common standards are required for evaluating outcome. For instance, many studies examine drug use only during the 30 days before the treatment is assessed. But is this really relevant for clinical purposes? Under what circumstances is a reduction in the number of days on which drugs are used an improvement – or is the wrong variable being measured? Clear notions about what criteria and what differences are really clinically relevant need to be developed.

Second, the research design should be clarified to improve its chances of producing clinically significant findings. The statistical power of the planned patient samples to detect a given difference in the outcome criterion of two treatments should be examined. The prerequisite is to estimate the true difference between treatment effects which is not usually known. Computer programmes are available to calculate such statistical power, such as 'Sample Power' in SPSS.

In pharmacological treatment, the ideal design is a placebo-controlled double-blind randomised study design, but in psychosocial treatment the situation is more complex. As for the methodological aspects of evaluation, the global aim is to control prospectively as many alternative influence variables as possible. In multi-site studies with large patient samples many such variables can be controlled in statistical analyses and the danger of unknown influence factors seems to be reduced, but, of course, not ruled out. The chances of natural studies producing meaningful findings without randomised treatment samples should be emphasised because in many cases it is not possible to randomise patients to different treatments.

Third, as mentioned above, meta-analytic studies provide more reliable and valid results than single studies and so should be carried out for different areas of interest. It would even be a step forward simply to count the number of studies with positive effects and those with no discernible or with negative effects. In the alcoholism field, Miller *et al.* (1995) demonstrated a very high correlation of 0.98 between this simple method and a complex index weighting the results according to qualitative criteria.

Finally, it seems necessary to develop complex models and theories, because reality does not consist of only two variables, one dependent and one independent. The literature reveals several models applying path analysis and structural equation models to the development of drug addiction (Taylor and Young, 1997). As a first step, any such models should be constructed as structural models (with knots or boxes as variables) closely related to empirical findings, but without structural equations.

Such mathematical functions are allocated to the variables in a second step followed by empirical analysis (e.g., by means of Linear Structural Relationship Analysis or LISREL) as a third step.

Systems theory and visualising techniques for developing models

Systems theory, not to be confused with systemic treatment, could provide the basis for model construction. It is a broad approach characterised by the following simple principles:

- A system is characterised by a number of aims or functions: a pile of sand is not a system unless it is a model for a landscape on a distinct scale. But a chair can be seen as a system: it has a function for the person sitting on it.
- A system is made up of a number of interconnected elements or subsystems.
- A system has a border to other systems. Thus the object's environment and affect on other objects around it need to be assessed.

Well-known principles of systems theory include the terms 'feedback' and 'regulation-system' to hold constant a variable such as the temperature in a room or the sugar level in the blood circulation system. Systems theory has several branches:

- general systems theory;
- cybernetics;
- black-box theory (Bischof, 1995); and
- simulation techniques for dynamic systems (Liebrand et al., 1998).

Visualising techniques are helpful tools for describing systems, their elements and relationships. At least two different notation systems can be distinguished (Küfner 1996, 1998):

- Within black-box analysis, arrows represent variables as input into or output from boxes. These boxes connect the input and output variables rather as rules or mathematical functions.
- Alternatively, and more important for structural equation models, arrows may mean only the influence of a variable represented as a knot (or box) to other knots or variables.

In another type of model describing the process of change, arrows symbolise a sequence of two time points related to the same variable without a causal relationship. An illustration of a graph model is given in Figure 2 below. Sometimes the different meanings of arrows, boxes and knots in diagrams are confusing and should be avoided. In structural equation models, knots or circles symbolise hypothetical constructs, which are assessed by operationalised variables.

In black-box analysis, influencing factors are analysed without knowing how the construct – for example, self-efficacy – is realised in the central nervous system. It may also be helpful to ask how the variables and their connecting boxes are realised in the biological system, leading to creative associations between psychosocial and

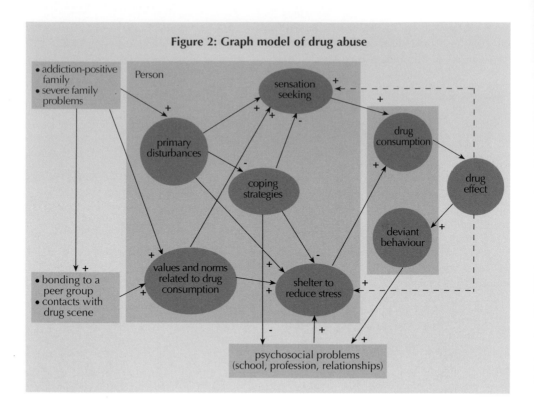

Figure 2: Graph model of drug abuse

biological perspectives. In the long term, an individual addiction model has to be based on biological systems, but without being reduced to biological processes.

Principles of systems theory should thus be combined with the development of a structural model – the first step in path analysis and in creating a structural equation model. Combining systems theory with computer-simulation techniques may also be beneficial. Such combinations could become powerful and useful tools in developing and testing models.

Strengths and shortcomings

In treatment settings, clinicians have to undertake concrete tasks to help patients to cope with their situation and to motivate them to change their unsuccessful behaviour. While clinicians thus know the problems inherent in treating individual cases better than researchers do, they are often too close to the patient and have problems formulating broader research questions not connected to the individual situation. If clinicians are interested in research findings and theoretical concepts they will also know the problems of applying those results to the individual case better than many researchers. The task here is not to comment on theoretical constructs such as motivation, but to aid evaluation research.

Clinicians tend to have limited knowledge about the principles of empirical research and research methodology. A simple overview of different types of evaluation can therefore help to differentiate the broad range of possible evaluation approaches.

Evaluation studies may examine the implementation of a programme, global and differential treatment outcomes, meta-analysis and cost–benefit analyses (Cartwright and Kaple, 1991). If clinicians understand these different types of evaluation – their benefits as well as their limitations – they will better understand the methods and results of empirical studies. One bridge between clinicians and researchers that still needs to be crossed is to define the standards of knowledge.

To ensure good-quality treatment, 'quality-control' measures are now being established in the addiction field. In Germany, this approach has been promoted primarily by health and pensions insurance companies, and only to a secondary degree by the treatment centres themselves.

Evaluation is a routine part of quality-control programmes and aims to discuss basic data within quality-control groups before deciding whether or not to make any changes in the treatment. Evaluation research should form the basis for evaluation procedures within quality-control measures. There is, therefore, a need to distinguish between quality control and evaluation research.

Figure 3: Overview of different forms of evaluation

1. Implementation:
   is the treatment programme feasible? Is its structure adequate for patients?

2. Global outcome (during treatment and at follow-up)

3. Treatment process interventions and patient behaviour:
   changes in patient variables

4. Differential outcome I:
   patient factors influencing outcome (patient variables as predictors)

5. Differential outcome II:
   treatment factors (as predictors) and outcome

6. Differential indication:
   interaction of patient and treatment variables

7. Meta-analysis of results in the literature

6. Cost–benefit study

Often, social trends are more influential than the results of evaluation studies. If no evaluation results are available, then interpretations and modern trends become the basis and background for deciding treatment characteristics. For example, treating male and female drug addicts together in one facility is not based on empirical findings, but on social trends. Indeed, some empirical results actually show that separate treatments for men and women produce better outcomes, at least for alcoholics (Küfner and Feuerlein, 1989).

Evaluation results and consequences

The treatment of drug addicts is working, but not very successfully. An indication of this is that the drop-out rates are frequently very high. In Germany, for example, about 70% of those undergoing in-patient drug-free rehabilitation terminate their treatment prematurely. In the literature, the drop-out rate is the strongest predictor (r = 0.3) of negative treatment outcome (Roch et al., 1992).

Likewise, the drop-out rate at a rehabilitation centre is an indicator of its treatment outcome with the advantage that it can be assessed within the treatment period without a cost-load catamnestic study. Clinicians and researchers may therefore focus on reducing the number of drop-outs and increasing time in treatment.

One new approach to reducing drop-out rates is a community-oriented treatment project in Germany based at a farm and involving minimal treatment (Vogt et al., 1995). Compared to the usual treatment with methadone or to in-patient rehabilitation this approach focuses on a new and totally different social environment with no illegal drugs and with no other clients present. Treatment is carried out as a counselling process between the individual client and the farmer's family. Since the influence of traditional psychotherapies on drug addicts is very limited, other forms of psychosocial influence could be helpful. Clinically oriented researchers could help identify different psychosocial approaches in a more systematic way.

At the same time, there should be a link to the pharmacological treatment approach. Presumably, both approaches are necessary and a combination of the two is probably more successful than a single approach (Ball and Ross, 1991). Analysing both psychosocial and pharmacological treatment evaluation research is thus indispensable.

Indication

One complex issue for clinicians that could benefit from research is that of indication. The empirical findings regarding indication in the field of drug addiction are, however, very poor, with, perhaps, one exception. Unlike with alcoholism, there is a widely accepted positive relationship between drug-treatment length and outcome. As to indication, McLellan (McLellan and Alterman, 1991) and others have shown that addicts suffering from the most severe problems achieve better results in longer-term treatments. This is not a very concrete strategy for indication, but it does demonstrate an empirical tendency.

Indication is not only a task of empirical evaluation research, and other aspects, such as costs, are equally important. Even without empirical knowledge about the differential effects of various treatments an indication strategy can be established.

The first indication strategy, in the case of no empirical findings about differential effects, is to apply minimal treatment. If this is not successful, the next intensive intervention should be applied.

The second strategy is always to apply the treatment that gives the best results. But in this case, the prerequisite is for an optimal treatment concept for all patients, which currently does not exist. It would thus be very unrealistic to attempt to apply this strategy. In cases which are not clear-cut, the tendency is to choose what is considered the best kind of treatment, whether or not this is really true, excluding cost aspects. Being certain of success seems to be more important than expense in this strategy.

The third indication strategy is oriented to the patients' special needs. If the patient has a problem in addition to the drug addiction – for example, a phobic disturbance – then additional treatment should be specified. This would seem to be a practical approach, if there are not too many additional disturbances requiring special treatment. The task of evaluation would be to show that this indicative treatment approach is more successful than a homogenous treatment concept for all drug addicts.

Finally, a fourth indication strategy applies the empirical results of evaluation studies to the effects of patient variables – such as age, gender, personality, co-morbidity – combined with treatment characteristics – for instance, treatment length, whether in-patient or outpatient, family treatment, interactional-oriented treatment or more social-skills treatment. An example of this approach is the MATCH project, which recently published its first, not very encouraging results of matching alcohol-dependent patients with treatment strategies (MATCH Research Group, 1997).

Considering these different strategies and the results of indication in evaluation studies, it can be said that evaluation studies and their results should be part of a more comprehensive approach or strategy for improving treatment.

Conclusions

The following suggestions could facilitate the transfer of information from research to clinical practice:

- In order to use evaluation results in a more intensive way, quality-control programmes should be established. These should be distinguished from evaluation research.

- A manual for using the results of evaluation studies should improve basic knowledge about evaluation methods and can help to assess studies and their results.

- By describing indication strategies it should be shown that empirical studies and their results may help to improve treatment if they are embedded in a comprehensive approach to optimise treatment. This means that clarifying the analysed treatment system and strategies are basic requirements for evaluation.

- Meta-analytic studies can summarise the growing number of empirical results.

- Using visualising techniques to construct models and formulate hypotheses can help to provide an overview of the complex relationships of influence variables.

- Systems theory for planning studies and structuring results can also be used to clarify relationships.

- Developing structural and causal models can help to connect theoretical constructs, measurement variables and evaluation results.

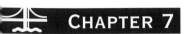

CHAPTER 7

TREATMENT INFORMATION SYSTEMS:
THE EMILIA-ROMAGNA EXPERIENCE

Umberto Nizzoli

The situation regarding treatment information systems in Reggio Emilia at the end of the 1980s could have been replicated in numerous other towns across Europe. At the time, numerous clinical forms existed, either developed in isolation, adapted from existing ones or copied from other services. As patients moved around and information was lost it became clear that such an *ad hoc* situation could not continue – everyone in one specific region needed to use the same forms.

In the Emilia area, articulating this need was a bottom-up process, which was accepted because the relationship between the health and social services and the regional government has always been a close one. At the same time, the Italian political and institutional infrastructure was grounded in the concept of 'subsidiarity', meaning that many competencies and powers were transferred in the early 1990s from the state to the regions, until a national health policy had all but disappeared.

Thus the Emilia-Romagna region, faced with taking responsibility for drug policy at regional level, needed as much reliable information on drug-treatment services and their clients as possible. A regional database form was thus developed to gather all possible information from drug misusers. The form was approved and all services operating in the region were obliged to use it. Since that time, no service has printed its own clinical forms.

The regional form is computerised, and every service has been provided with the relevant hardware, software and training to use it. Each participating service also has its own database staff, co-ordinated by a network known as the Observatory Group. As a result, the Emilia-Romagna region can now provide information about its service users that is unparalleled in Italy.

Difficulties, however, still remain. As it is now some time since the forms were first developed, the problem has arisen of incorporating unforeseen data streams. As before, even in services long used to completing database forms, staff must also be constantly encouraged, reminded and cajoled to use them. Moreover, the forms are sometimes rejected at the service level itself. In one case, a service chose not to receive funds rather than comply with the terms and conditions of data delivery.

This non-compliance is sometimes caused by unnecessary demands for data not included on the forms at state level. Some services, therefore, do not supply data to the Departments of Internal Affairs or Health. Of Italy's 560 such services, only 480–90 send their data to government departments. A final reason for the opposition to using the forms is that the region reserves the right to make the information provided public. For instance, it compares the services and draws up a 'league table' of the best and the worst.

TedEval: a simple evaluation technique

In the early 1990s, the region's Psychotherapy Group began to search for an instrument which could be used to measure treatment effectiveness *during* a course of treatment rather than only at its end. The Addiction Severity Index (ASI) was deemed unsuitable, and other sources were examined in 1993 and 1994. From this extensive search, a unique instrument was created.

First, treatment outcomes were defined, with consensus reached on the meaning of each and every one. Similar outcomes were grouped together, and a hierarchy drawn up. From this list, what was believed to be the most suitable database form was defined. The final result contained 20 items covering six areas of client observation:

- physical status;
- mental functioning;
- relationship status;
- social conditions;
- judicial status; and
- drug consumption.

This instrument, called TedEval, describes the seriousness of the patient's status using a score from 0–1,000. It is designed for use at intake (usually after the third interview) and should be repeated after six months to detect any possible changes. TedEval is confidential and reliable, and is also easy to complete (taking about seven minutes). As such, it is perfectly compatible with a service's clinical activities. The reading of the data contained within TedEval enables agency staff to consider the merits of the therapeutic strategy being applied.

Although some practitioners argued for the production of a manual to accompany TedEval, none was produced, both for reasons of time and to give the practitioner the opportunity to make his or her own subjective interpretations. Guidelines were, however, provided on the use of the instrument. As virtually every service held a weekly meeting to discuss the clients' case histories, it was recommended that TedEval become a regular part of this meeting, allowing solutions to be defined that were best suited to the individual's needs.

After a trial period of more than two years involving many hundreds of cases, TedEval has demonstrated itself to be a useful *subjective* indicator, with responsibility for its effectiveness ultimately lying with the group that uses it. As such, TedEval is a vital instrument in the weekly discussion that takes place in every operational group.

The Psychotherapy Group is researching the evolution of TedEval in 11 hospital centres, and a validation study is currently in progress. There is now a computerised TedEval which is even simpler to use, taking just 2–3 minutes to complete. An artificial-intelligence system of neural networks has been 'taught' to give a certain score to each answer for each item, and therefore provides an on-screen profile of the strengths and weaknesses of each patient. This computerised instrument can also give a final score from 0–1,000. The possible range of drug use has been divided into six stages: light use (under 180); medium–light (180–279); medium (280–479); medium–serious (480–599); serious (600–779); and very serious (780–1,000).

Emilia-Romagna's evaluation system

While Emilia-Romagna's Psychotherapy Group has been developing this evaluation instrument, the Observatory Group has co-ordinated the various related databases. Although the former group focuses on changes in the individual patient, the latter concentrates on the effectiveness of the regional service as a whole. As a consequence, database items such as 'number of overdose deaths' or 'percentage of sero-conversions' can become important indicators of the work carried out at regional level.

The Observatory Group has developed a self-complete instrument to measure clients' consumption of various substances, the rationale being that a reduction in the level of drug use is thought to be the fundamental indicator motivating the existence of drug services and ensuring their effectiveness. The Italian version of the Nottingham Health Profile is also used to measure client well-being.

These two questionnaires, in conjunction with TedEval (and another questionnaire on customer satisfaction developed by the Group of Warrantors), represent the treatment-evaluation package – weighted towards the 'client' as 'customer' – currently used in Emilia-Romagna.

ERIT: the multi-disciplinary and multi-national perspective of evaluation

It can no longer be said that treatment evaluation in Europe is lacking. Of course, taking Europe as a whole, it is still scant, applied only by a minority of drug services. However, each EU Member State has undertaken important treatment-evaluation exercises and, although irregular, evaluation is increasing. Crucial to this development is the need for inter- and intra-sectoral communication.

ERIT, the Federation of European Professionals Working in the Field of Drug Abuse, is just such a forum for communication and sharing evaluative experiences. Already, the Federation has collected some 20 different evaluation instruments which will soon be published to promote good practice.

The key to all these instruments, whether large or small, is validation. Since many instruments have not been rigorously tested, an organisation like ERIT can provide a 'meta-validation' by comparing instruments. The goal of ERIT's evaluation project, therefore, is not to champion one particular instrument or to develop new techniques; it is simply to synthesise (so as better to share) experiences. The project is also designed to spread the culture of evaluation, through monographs, seminars and conferences.

One of the key issues identified through ERIT's evaluation work is the importance of the institutional, judicial and social contexts in which treatment evaluation is carried out. Not only does the meaning of evaluation derive from the context, but also the significance and scores attributed to that evaluation. This recognition should encourage a redoubling of efforts to work towards creating a social Europe, the fundamental condition for the spread of common evaluation instruments.

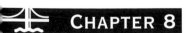 CHAPTER 8

TREATMENT EVALUATION IN THE UK: THE NATIONAL TREATMENT OUTCOME RESEARCH STUDY

Michael Gossop, John Marsden, Duncan Stewart, Petra Lehmann, Carolyn Edwards, Alison Wilson, Graham Segar

The National Treatment Outcome Research Study (NTORS) is a large-scale, multi-site, prospective study of treatment outcome conducted with a cohort of more than 1,000 drug users who entered treatment services in England in 1995. The study was specifically commissioned by the UK government to provide evidence of the effectiveness of existing drug-misuse treatment services.

NTORS is the largest study of drug-treatment outcome ever conducted in the UK, although similar large-scale investigations have been conducted in the United States. These US studies include the Drug Abuse Reporting Program (DARP – Simpson and Sells, 1990), the Treatment Outcome Prospective Study (TOPS – Hubbard *et al.*, 1989) and the 'six cities' research on methadone maintenance (Ball and Ross, 1991). Such research has demonstrated that treating drug problems can be effective. However, the difficulty of generalising from studies carried out in other countries is considerable as the characteristics of drug abuse and of drug abusers will differ in many respects from country to country, as will the types of treatment provided.

Studies of the type and scale of NTORS are costly. They are expensive both in financial terms and in terms of the scientific and human resources required. They also rely on serious and sustained commitment from many individuals and organisations. Prospective outcome studies are, therefore, rare. It is partly for these reasons that no such investigation has previously been carried out in the UK.

The further significance of NTORS is in part due to the fact that it has been designed and implemented as a *national* study, investigating treatment programmes from all over England. It is also a *large-scale* study with a *comprehensive* design, looking in detail at the social and psychological characteristics of clients, as well as at a wide range of treatment operational factors in relation to multiple measures of treatment outcome. For these reasons, the results of NTORS will contribute to the scientific understanding of treatment outcome and will provide valuable data about the impact of national treatment responses on drug problems. If the effectiveness of treatment interventions for drug problems is to be improved, policy-makers, researchers, service purchasers and providers all need to have a clearer understanding of the many factors that contribute to the success or otherwise of treatment, so that drug services and interventions can be developed and strengthened.

NTORS includes detailed and empirically based information about the pre-treatment behaviours, problems and social circumstances of the cohort, and the operational characteristics of the treatment programmes and interventions. As part of the research project, it will provide economic cost-estimates for the problems associated with drug abuse among the NTORS cohort. Most importantly, it will provide a detailed account of the impact of treatment in terms of the clinically significant psychological, social and behavioural changes that are observed.

Research design and methodology

NTORS monitors the progress of clients newly recruited into one of four treatment modalities:

- specialist in-patient units;
- residential rehabilitation services;
- methadone-maintenance programmes; and
- methadone-reduction programmes.

The term 'modality' is used to refer to a broad category of treatment intervention. Within this category it is accepted that there may be some (possibly considerable) degree of variation. However, the treatment interventions included within each modality should have general defining characteristics and common features, such as the treatment setting within which the intervention is provided, the goals of treatment or the types of procedures followed.

The study's research design is based on a tradition of programme evaluation and longitudinal outcome research developed in the United States. It is naturalistic, and causal inference is achieved by measuring key variables and comparing treatment samples on the basis of pre- and post-treatment outcome measures. This design was chosen in preference to a randomised control design, as the client's own baseline measures in NTORS are used as a control condition to assess change. In a naturalistic or quasi-experimental design such as that employed in this case, pre-existing differences in client characteristics, as well as differences in social and environmental circumstances, may explain some of the outcome variations across programmes. NTORS measures such differences so that they can be taken into account when examining which factors influenced what outcomes.

Services of potential usefulness to NTORS were selected after considering:

- the capacity of the specific agency and, in particular, its ability to recruit a sufficient number of cases within the restricted time available – 'capacity' was defined in terms of the number of new cases presenting to the agency in the last month (at least 20 estimated new clients); and

- the location of the service – NTORS required agencies which were located throughout the health regions of England, but which were also based in areas with a representative prevalence of drug problems and drug-treatment services.

A total of 54 agencies were selected:

- 16 methadone-maintenance programmes;
- 15 methadone-reduction programmes;
- 15 residential rehabilitation services; and
- eight specialist in-patient units.

After participation in the project had been agreed, NTORS researchers visited all the agencies involved. The purpose of these visits was to familiarise and train drug workers in the use of the Maudsley Addiction Profile (MAP) interview procedures (see below). Training manuals were also left at each agency for future reference. In addition, these visits allowed the necessary administrative procedures to be set up to ensure that agencies would be in regular contact with the two research bases (London and Manchester). Researchers encouraged a named individual at each agency to take responsibility for the on-site co-ordination of the project. Finally, these centres were provided with posters and leaflets to advertise the study to their clients.

The Maudsley Addiction Profile

The Maudsley Addiction Profile is a set of structured research interviews developed specifically for the NTORS project. The MAP profiles the social circumstances, key problems and experiences of drug users not only at entry into treatment, but also at the follow up points during and after leaving treatment. The MAP interviews have been designed so that the key NTORS measures are repeatedly assessed during and after treatment, allowing the study to assess the impact of the particular treatment modality. The information needs of NTORS have been carefully balanced against the burden on staff time in interviewing clients, and so the MAP has been designed to be used by clinical and agency staff without formal research training.

There were three stages to the MAP's development.

- First, an initial pool of measures was compiled. These items included substance use and drug risk-taking behaviours, physical and psychological health, criminal involvement and social functioning (relationships, employment, education and training, etc.). A further set of measures was incorporated concerning the psychological aspects of drug use, motivation for treatment and coping strategies. These items may be useful for understanding the manner in which clients respond to treatment, as well as to longer-term recovery.

- Second, draft versions of the MAP interviews were piloted with samples of drug users in several treatment services. This led to further refinements and improvements in item structure and interview design, and two specific modifications were made. On the basis of the feedback from pilot interviews, a response-card booklet was prepared to assist interview completion for each of the six MAP instruments. This has several benefits. It makes the interview quicker and easier to complete, enhancing interviewee attention. It also assists confidentiality in different settings since the respondent can read the number of an item rather than the item itself. Another design modification concerned questions about involvement in criminal activity and with the criminal-justice system. Given the sensitivity of this topic, the respondent was given the option of using a self-complete questionnaire for this section of the interview.

- Third, a training strategy was implemented by the NTORS team to help agency staff administer the MAP interviews. Instruction manuals were prepared describing the rationale and structure of the interviews with detailed notes on the interview procedure and item completion. The research team then conducted on-site training sessions for staff at each centre to ensure familiarity with the MAP. Subsequent feedback suggested that this procedure was valuable both as a specific learning exercise and for enhancing working links between NTORS and treatment staff. A pack of materials was prepared for each participating agency containing information for clients, consent forms, the MAP interviews and response cards, and enrolment forms. A single 'at-a-glance' information sheet was also designed for the treatment staff, outlining the procedure to be followed for client enrolment and completion of the MAP-1 interview.

The MAP-1 is a structured interview of about 45 minutes' duration. It has seven sections:

- background information;
- drug and alcohol use;
- change, motivation and coping;
- health;
- relationships;
- legal issues; and
- treatment.

Six scales which have been used in previous research were selected and adapted to assess issues 2–7. A full description of the development of these measures is available from the authors.

The MAP scales will facilitate comparison of NTORS data with previous research. Some new items were developed specifically for the study, particularly within the legal and treatment sections. The legal section of the MAP looks in detail at involvement with the criminal-justice system and criminal activity. The treatment section records the client's treatment history and use of hospital, residential and community services for medical, psychological and substance-use problems. Successive MAP interviews administered during and after the index treatment episode comprise a core set of repeated measures from the above domains.

National treatment modalities

The four types of treatment modality within NTORS included residential and out-patient- or community-based treatments. The two residential treatments were specialist in-patient units and residential rehabilitation services. The two community or outpatient treatments were programmes providing either maintenance or reduction with methadone (or with other substitute drugs).

In-patient units

The UK's specialist in-patient drug-dependence units (DDUs) were established in the late 1960s, and in many respects the system is unique to that country. In-patient units are typically located within a psychiatric hospital and provide medically supervised detoxification coupled with counselling and support interventions. Usually, in-patient programmes are staffed – and treatment delivered – by multidisciplinary teams, although psychiatric, medical and nursing staff are the most common members of such teams. Programmes may vary in length from about two weeks to a maximum of three months, and there are relatively few specialist in-patient DDUs in the UK with this treatment approach.

Residential rehabilitation

Residential services include those run by a number of large national bodies. An important and influential recent development is the growth of Twelve-Step and Minnesota Model programmes, directed towards recovery through abstinence. Unlike the in-patient units, many residential programmes are located away from inner-city areas in order to provide a clear change of setting. Typically, abstinence is a treatment goal, although these programmes vary widely in terms of treatment philosophy. In the UK, the four main types of residential rehabilitation are the Twelve-Step programmes, Therapeutic Communities, Christian Houses and General Houses. Some residential projects manage detoxification directly, but most require addicts to be drug-free on admission. Treatment length varies from short-term with aftercare to long-term programmes of over one year.

Methadone maintenance

Since the establishment of UK drug clinics in the late 1960s, maintenance treatment has usually been delivered by specialist services, although more recently methadone treatment can also be delivered by General Practitioners, either independently or in association with a specialist drug agency – the so-called 'shared care' model. British methadone maintenance differs from the US model in that the methadone is often offered to the addict via a prescription which is taken to a retail chemist. The pharmacist then dispenses the drug to the patient, which is typically consumed without supervision. The drug is prescribed from the outset on a stable-dose, non-reducing basis. Following stabilisation at a suitable dose, the client may be maintained for either a fixed or an indefinite period.

In addition to this traditional British method of prescribing maintenance drugs, in recent years there has been an increase in 'American-style' methadone maintenance in which clients attend a clinic each day and take their drugs under supervision. This has sometimes been referred to in the UK as 'structured methadone maintenance'. Eight such programmes were established as pilot projects by the Department of Health in 1995 and these programmes and their clients are included in NTORS.

Methadone reduction

Methadone-reduction programmes can be regarded as abstinence-oriented interventions and, where they provide short-term reduction within a period of less than 6–8 weeks, they may also be regarded as detoxification programmes. Methadone-reduction programmes are likely to vary in duration from periods of a few weeks to many months, possibly even years. Alterations may be made to the implementation of dose reductions or the duration of the treatment because of changed circumstances or crises presented by the client. In practice, many UK agencies operate a mixture of methadone-reduction and maintenance responses.

NTORS clients and their problems

Agency staff approached all eligible clients starting treatment between 27 February and 31 July 1995 and invited them to participate in NTORS. Clients were eligible for an intake interview providing that all the following criteria were met:

- they were starting a new treatment episode;
- they presented with a drug-related problem (other than alcohol);
- they were able to provide an address in the UK for follow-up; and
- they were not a previous client of NTORS.

Overall, 1,110 eligible clients were recruited over the five-month period. Since 35 did not provide sufficient locator information to allow follow-up, the sample base was revised down to 1,075.

Table 1: Clients recruited into NTORS by treatment type

Treatment type	Number of clients recruited	% of cohort
In-patient	122	11.3
Residential rehabilitation	286	26.6
Methadone maintenance	458	42.6
Methadone reduction	209	19.4

Table 2: Demographic profile at treatment entry

Characteristic	In-patient	Residential	Methadone maintenance	Methadone reduction
	(n = 122)	(n = 286)	(n = 458)	(n = 209)
Male (%)	77	74	72	73
Female (%)	23	26	28	27
Mean age (years)	30	29	30	27
White (%)	94	88	90	93

The largest number of clients were recruited from the methadone-maintenance programmes. This was mainly due to the inclusion of the eight pilot structured methadone-maintenance projects within the NTORS framework, which contributed 350 recruits to the study.

At the point of entry to treatment, only 127 (11.8%) of the client group reported having a job, 89% had been unemployed in the previous three months and the majority (81%) reported being 'mostly unemployed' during the past two years.

Most of the cohort were multiple or polydrug users. Few restricted their use to one drug, although dependence on heroin was the single most common drug problem, and the average length of heroin use for the cohort was nine years (s.d. = 5.8 years). The relative severity of the drug-abuse problems experienced by the NTORS clients must therefore be borne in mind when evaluating the impact of treatment.

In the three-month period before starting NTORS treatment, there was frequent benzodiazepine use among the cohort. While approximately one in five clients were using benzodiazepines every day, a further one in six were using regularly each week and another one in six on an occasional basis. For some clients, benzodiazepine use will be licit, prescribed by a physician for a psychological disorder, and this prescription may or may not be misused by the patient. Others, particularly the occasional users, were taking these drugs illicitly – particularly diazepam and temazepam.

An important finding was that the frequency of crack cocaine use was *higher* than that of cocaine powder in every frequency-of-use category. Forty-nine people used crack every day in the three months before intake, a further 130 (12%) were regular weekly users and 199 reported using crack less than weekly. It was rare for the NTORS cohort to be daily users of cocaine powder: only 1% used daily, although 17% used on an occasional or weekly basis.

Overall, 62% of the cohort reported that they had injected a drug in the three months prior to treatment. There were no statistically significant differences between men and women, nor between treatment modalities. The usual route of administration was intravenous for 59% of the clients who had used heroin in the three months prior to treatment, while 40% of heroin users smoked the drug. Cocaine powder and amphetamines were also frequently injected – approximately half of those who had used these drugs in the previous three months had injected them.

During the three months prior to treatment, 156 clients (14.5%) reported using a needle or syringe after someone else had used it, and there was a higher rate of pre-treatment needle and syringe sharing amongst female drug users. This pattern of needle sharing has been observed in clinical populations and may indicate sharing between sexual partners. Sharing rates also differed significantly across treatment modality, with clients in residential treatment being more likely to report having used a needle or syringe after somebody else had done so.

Shoplifting was the most commonly reported illegal activity, with more than one-third of the cohort having committed at least one such offence in the three months before intake. Fraud and burglary were also quite common, and more than one-quarter reported selling drugs. Almost three-quarters of the full cohort had been arrested in the two years before intake (again, most commonly for shoplifting, although about one-third had been arrested for a drug offence). There were differences in the criminal-activity profile of clients entering the various treatment modalities.

Similar differences were found for treatment contact, although the treatment histories typically reveal multiple help-seeking from different drug-treatment services. Rates of previous psychiatric treatment were highest for the residential and in-patient clients. A higher proportion of drug users entering the in-patient and residential modalities had received past hospital psychiatric treatment when compared to the community methadone programmes (in-patient: 14%; residential: 15%; methadone maintenance: 8%; methadone reduction: 6%). Clients in residential programmes were also more likely to have received community psychiatric treatment (21%) and to report receiving treatment from an Accident and Emergency department (64%).

Current project status

NTORS is still at a comparatively early stage. Analyses of the available six-month and 12-month data are being conducted, and reports on both six- and 12-month outcome are currently in preparation. Initial results show substantial improvements in all the target problem behaviours immediately after starting treatment. Specific improvements have been noted in the use of heroin and other illicit drugs, and there have also been reductions in injecting and needle sharing. Criminal behaviour has dropped and measures of physical and psychological health show further improvements. Summaries of these results are in the public domain (see Gossop et al., 1996, 1997).

Preliminary analyses suggest that outcomes followed up after six months are likely to be broadly similar to those at the earlier follow-up point and to show substantial improvements in most key outcome measures. In particular, there are marked reductions in the use of illicit opiates including heroin, as well as in the use of other drugs, such as cocaine and amphetamines. These and other results became available in 1997, although they were unavailable at the time of writing. Funding for NTORS will allow the clients to continue to be followed up into the next century.

TREATMENT EVALUATION AND POLICY

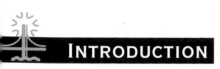

PART III

INTRODUCTION

*I*n this final section, the impact of treatment evaluation on policy-makers (local, European and international) is discussed.

In Chapter 9, Elfriede Koller draws upon her experiences co-ordinating drug policy at ministerial level in the German Länder. The lack of evaluation research is a source of frustration for policy- and decision-makers, leaving them open to the influence of 'opinion-makers' rather than scientific evidence. With little or no comparative evaluation and no definition of what constitutes 'success', Koller argues, the financing of many treatment programmes relies on little more than goodwill and faith. Treatment evaluation and inter-sectoral co-operation and co-ordination are therefore vital if the correct decisions are to be made.

In Chapter 10, Ambros Uchtenhagen provides an overview of the European Union's COST A-6 programme on treatment evaluation (Evaluation of Action against Drug Abuse in Europe). The programme's main objectives are to establish networks of researchers at national and international level, to collect and analyse relevant research material, to develop protocols and instruments for evaluation research and to stimulate international multi-site evaluation research. Over its five-year lifespan, the programme has developed the European Addiction Severity Index (EuropASI) evaluation instrument, as well as the Treatment Unit Form for gathering information on drug-treatment services. It has also reviewed the relevant European evaluation studies, the instruments and methodologies employed by those studies, and built a European network of scientists and professionals engaged in evaluation research so that information may be exchanged, workshops run and guidelines on treatment evaluation prepared.

In Chapter 11, Maristela Monteiro describes the role of the World Health Organisation's Programme on Substance Abuse (WHO/PSA). Urging consideration for cost effectiveness, Monteiro argues for educating policy- and decision-makers – as well as programme-managers – in the need for evaluation. An appreciation of the benefits of, and the need for, proper evaluation must be developed before evaluation can be fully accepted and implemented on a regular basis. The WHO vision of the value of treatment evaluation is founded on the belief that planning and delivering specific treatments should be based on a careful analysis of needs, competing demands, knowledge of the relative cost-effectiveness of alternative means of delivering services and the explicit recognition of the scarcity of resources and the need for maximum efficiency in the way they are used.

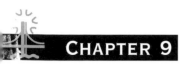

CHAPTER 9

THE POLICY-MAKER'S PERSPECTIVE

Elfriede Koller

In Germany, the number of treatment facilities for drug abusers has increased in the last few years, as treatment is generally considered the most effective way of reducing drug-related problems. Having been told that 'no two drug users are the same', the diversification of treatment received the full support of national decision-makers. Treatments targeted at drug-dependent women, families and ethnic minorities were all encouraged, as were short-term, long-term, in- and outpatient treatments. Low-threshold units were also created and maintenance programmes came to be seen as crucial.

However, despite the vast sums invested in the diversification of treatment, most of the decisions to fund such treatment modalities were not based on scientific evidence and did not lead to results any better than the 'rule of thirds': one-third of clients achieve abstinence; one-third improve, but are not abstinent; and one-third make no progress.

Since their establishment, some of the new approaches have been evaluated, but again, in many cases, this assessment has been found to have little scientific basis – all too often, the new project was found to be 'essential' only as a means of ensuring future funding. As far as this author is aware, no published evaluation research has found that the treatment being assessed is of no benefit at all to its clients.

Fundamentally, and until very recently, no-one has even been able to compare one treatment with another to see what is 'successful', nor has there been any comparative evaluation of short-term versus long-term treatment. Governments therefore finance this broad range of diverse treatment approaches in order to offer different choices to different people – even though the success of this variety of options remains unproven.

Policy- and decision-makers clearly suffer from this lack of accurate evidence, and end up being buffeted by the forces of 'opinion-makers', rather than being guided by scientific research. The problem, of course, is that national drug policy depends on a wide variety of interests and influences, such as public opinion and media pressure to come up with innovative and effective ways to tackle the threat of drug abuse.

The interests of treatment centres to survive, of clients to have the most individual and accessible route into treatment, and of insurance companies that pay for such treatment and have their own philosophy of standards, costs and outcomes must also be weighed up. While these pragmatic aspects are rarely considered by researchers undertaking treatment evaluation, for better or worse, they do play a central role for decision-makers.

The need for robust treatment evaluation

Drug treatment in Germany is generally considered to be of high quality. Evaluation is of the utmost importance in this system, but the questions asked are no longer simply whether an effect occurs or not or whether a programme is 'good' or 'successful'. Instead, evaluation today is linked to supporting objective-oriented development. This is because there has been a fundamental change in the way treatment is perceived in Germany.

National care systems are no longer thought of institutionally, but in terms of the functions they should fulfil and the client needs they are expected to satisfy. This new perspective changes the way in which the individual parties providing help in the health-care system co-operate with one another: co-operation is changing from an essentially static form to a dynamic, goal-oriented one. As a result, evaluation now has to focus on the function of assistance, not on the institution providing that help.

Meanwhile, 'productivity', 'quality', 'efficacy' and 'outcome' are all common terms within drug-treatment centres. But these terms alone do not make a treatment. In order to provide the right help to the right people, the demand for successful co-ordination and co-operation needs to be placed within the context of local monitoring and steering. In other words, evaluation needs to be seen as more significant than simply a means of representing and assessing treatment conditions and performance.

Within this model, evaluation has the task of finding the most effective form of care for a particular client at a particular time. Even now, such a requirement is not deemed to be an important factor in scientific evaluation – but it will clearly become a vital issue in the future.

If evaluation cannot answer this most basic of questions – what treatment is best suited to which client? – the drug-care system has no future at all. Instead, family doctors, social services, psychiatric institutions and rehabilitation clinics could well take over the care of drug users.

The need for inter-sectoral co-operation and co-ordination

In Germany, the distinction between care for those addicted to legal drugs and those addicted to illegal drugs is becoming blurred. These two fields of care developed in almost complete isolation, but the lines of separation are now being increasingly questioned.

With the more integrative perspective described above, policy- and decision-makers are realising that few drug misusers actually follow the 'classic career'. As such, addicts are no longer considered as a population that should be cordoned off from the general public. The effectiveness of creating such 'enclaves' is disputed, and health and social services that cater to the general population are now being urged to open their doors and meet the requirements of drug addicts. The expectation is that intra- and, above all, *inter*-sectoral co-operation will improve, leading to a more effective provision of help to those addicted.

Given this situation, evaluation research should now examine the question of inter-sectoral co-operation. This term refers to concept-controlled, objective-oriented co-ordination between public bodies, private institutions, networks and helping services.

The care system

The current care system for drug addicts in Germany is made up of the following three sectors.

- *Sector I* is specifically for drug addicts and abusers, and provides special advice centres and clinics. As stated at the beginning of this chapter, within the last decade, this sector has expanded and 'traditional' drug-based treatments are now enhanced by low-threshold services, street work, harm-reduction and damage-control techniques.

- *Sector II* provides psycho-social and psychiatric aid within public, social and health-care institutions. This sector deals with 'difficult' cases, clients not motivated to change and chronic addicts.

- *Sector III* is the basic medical system, encompassing physicians, family doctors and general hospitals. Most drug addicts are treated – initially at least – within this sector, but in general, the medical sector has little competence in the specific area of addiction, as all the public money for drug care tends to go to Sector I.

This fragmentation and lack of co-ordination means that the system as a whole leans towards institution-related thought and action. The resultant tendency is to select clients according to the criteria of the particular institution. This creates a situation in which Sector I cannot adequately satisfy the requirements of chronic addicts. The irony is that the clients requiring the most help – who will have complex social and health problems which cannot be tackled effectively by a psychiatrist – as a rule receive the least assistance.

The needs of the policy-maker

All the above reinforces the need for better inter-sectoral co-operation and co-ordination, issues which should concern any future evaluation. This requirement also implies that evaluation research must focus both on treatment systems as a whole and on the individual case.

A 'community system' consists of various agencies, care and treatment settings, providing both specialist and generic services. Evaluation should examine the impact of these agencies and services on individual clients and monitor their progress across a range of objectives. As far as this author is aware, systematic research is not carried out at these two apparently opposite ends of the spectrum – the treatment system and the individual.

Decision-makers want to learn what benefits clients can receive from a given drug-care system, and what type of client has what specific need. In short, they want a client-oriented picture, not an institution-oriented one. At this policy level, evaluating the 'success' of a single service is therefore not the primary objective. On the other hand, regional treatment systems can only be planned or restructured if community systems are evaluated.

Recommendations for future action

This chapter has sought to show that evaluation needs to become a tool to promote structures and systems according to specific goals. It has also stressed the urgent need to evaluate inter-sectoral co-operation, a task that would require new concepts and definitions.

New concepts

To start with, the status quo would need to be analysed and the following questions addressed:

- How many people require specific interventions for certain addiction-related problems?
- What institutions with what resources offer what type of help for what type of problem?
- Which clients with what problems will be reached by those offers of help?

Such an analysis of a given situation will provide an initial picture of the 'helping network', including the co-operative relationships within and between the different care sectors. The evaluation also has to distinguish between the two types of co-operation: institution-related co-operation; and client-related co-operation.

An analysis at this level will uncover the strengths and weaknesses as well as the advantages and disadvantages of existing collaboration. The following questions should be posed:

- What overlaps and deficiencies are there in the provision of individual care?
- Have personal responsibilities been made clear to the clients and if so how has this been done?
- Has information exchange and co-operation been formal or informal?

- At what levels does co-operation take place and in what form?
- Are offers of treatment agreed and measures co-ordinated, and if so how is this done?
- Are joint activities planned and carried out?
- Are resources used jointly?
- Do institutional links exist?
- What weak points of co-operation and co-ordination can be identified?

Client-related co-operation

Client-related co-operation should also be investigated, and this investigation should be carried out in a standardised and qualitative manner. The following parameters should be recorded:

- the goal and type of aid;
- the continuity of the provision of help in terms of personnel and concept;
- the participating workers;
- the type of client information shared or exchanged with other professionals;
- the frequency and form of such information exchanges;
- the scale and nature of co-ordination of the assistance provided to the client; and
- client participation.

This investigation should assist in developing recommendations for improving the effectiveness and efficacy of an observed network or care system.

Data collection

Within the framework of inter-sectoral co-operation, data must be collected in a manner that allows comparisons to be made and the 'treatment trail' to be followed. For conclusions to be drawn about the relationship between the care system and the use that clients make of it, while respecting client confidentiality, the clients need to be identifiable, at least in coded form.

Professional views

Finally, drug workers themselves can provide useful information on certain issues which improve or hinder their work. A worker questionnaire should therefore be prepared to collect information on professional and 'ideological' views, as well as on possible areas of competition for clients and resources. This analysis should concentrate on areas where either obvious differences or common ground can be perceived.

The role of the EMCDDA

With the European Monitoring Centre for Drugs and Drug Addiction supporting the above procedures, there would at last be more – and better – evaluation which could reinforce and intensify the monitoring of the treatment process according to its over-all goals. The ultimate goal must be that such a targeted evaluation could uncover hitherto unseen relationships within an overall treatment system, leading to a policy or strategy which could make the entire experience fruitful for both the care system and its clients.

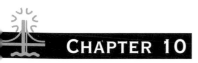

CHAPTER 10

COST A-6's Contribution to Treatment Evaluation

Ambros Uchtenhagen

Since the early 1990s, European Co-operation and Co-ordination in the Field of Scientific and Technical Research among European Union and European Free Trade Association Countries (COST) has developed research programmes in ten areas of the social sciences. Drug abuse is one of these ten areas.

COST A-6, Evaluation of Action against Drug Abuse in Europe, was established on the initiative of a group with differing interests. This explains its diverse working programme that focuses on the evaluation not only of drug policy, but also of primary prevention, treatment, rehabilitation and action against drug-related delinquency.

The programme ran from December 1992 to December 1997 with the collaboration of 15 European countries and invited observers from the Commission of the European Union, the United Nations International Drug Control Programme (UNDCP), the World Health Organisation (WHO) European office and the Pompidou Group of the Council of Europe. It also established links with a number of European professional associations – the European Federation of Therapeutic Communities, ITACA and the Federation of European Professionals Working in the Field of Drug Abuse (ERIT) – and research groups – such as the Social Science Research Group on Drug Dependence, the International Study on Drug Treatment Systems and the European Association on Substance Abuse Research.

The main objectives of COST-A6 were to:

- establish networks of researchers at national and international level;
- collect and analyse relevant research material;
- develop protocols and instruments for evaluation research; and
- stimulate international multi-site evaluation research.

Protocols and instruments

A working group was also set up to develop research protocols and instruments. Chaired by Anna Kokkevi and Ambros Uchtenhagen, this group focused primarily on developing a client information system, selecting from the available instruments the Addiction Severity Index (ASI) and adapting it to European conditions. A manual for using the European Addiction Severity Index (EuropASI) was published in 1995 (Blanken *et al.*, 1995). Translations are now available in Dutch, English, Finnish, French, German, Greek, Italian, Russian and Spanish, while versions of EuropASI in other languages are currently being prepared.

The validity of EuropASI was initially assessed within the framework of a co-morbidity study co-ordinated by Anna Kokkevi, and guidelines for validation studies in various other countries are also being developed. Training courses for EuropASI have been held in Belgium, Germany, Greece, Italy and the Netherlands. A final workshop was run in collaboration with the European Addiction Training Institute in November 1997.

The second aim of this working group was to identify a similar instrument for gathering information on drug-treatment services. As none of the existing instruments were deemed to satisfy every need, the group developed its own Treatment Unit Form (TUF), a preliminary version of which is now being piloted by the EMCDDA. The results of this study will inform the group's future work.

National funding has also helped in developing systems to monitor treatment services. In Stockholm, V. Segraeus has developed another model for gathering information on drug treatment, while in Zurich, S. Schaaf has carried out a comprehensive review of all treatment-information models and instruments as the basis for conceptualising a modular instrument to describe substance-abuse treatment (MIDES).

Treatment evaluation

Alongside the working group developing research protocols and instruments sat another group – chaired by M. Coletti – to examine the evaluation of drug treatment. This group's objectives were to:

- review relevant European evaluation studies;
- review the methodology and instruments used in such studies; and
- build a European network of scientists and professionals engaged in evaluation research, so that information can be exchanged, workshops run and guidelines on treatment evaluation prepared.

The group commissioned country reports from Belgium, France, Germany, Greece, Italy, the Netherlands, Norway, Portugal, Spain, Sweden, Switzerland and the UK which summarised the results, focus and methodology of evaluation studies already carried out in these countries. The reports revealed an extremely diverse picture of treatment evaluation, reflecting not only different treatment systems, but also different research priorities. Whereas follow-up studies of individual treatment programmes were the norm in most countries, others – most notably Germany, Norway, Switzerland and the UK – had made considerable efforts to develop systematic client-documentation and treatment-evaluation systems on a national basis.

Germany has two national documentation systems: EBIS for out-patient treatment (set up in 1980); and SEDOS for in-patient treatment (set up in 1994). In Switzerland, there are four such systems – SAMBAD for out-patients (1996), SAKRAM for in-patient alcoholics (1992), FOS for in-patient drug misusers (1996) and PROVE for prescribing narcotics (1994). SAMBAD, FOS and PROVE are largely compatible with each other and with EuropASI. The UK currently has one national documentation system, the Maudsley Addiction Profile (MAP), for in- and out-patients (1995, see Chapter 8 above) and a national system is currently under construction in Norway.

Based on an analysis of the country reports, the working group produced a paper which reviewed the various national documentation systems as a basis for comparative evaluation.

The group has also commissioned a number of studies on specific aspects of treatment-evaluation methodology. For researchers, the focus has been on outcome evaluation; for practitioners, on process evaluation; and for administrators, on cost–benefit analysis. Adequate instruments for process evaluation and cost–benefit analysis have yet to be identified and developed.

Based on the group's work on methodological issues – as well as a number of other recent studies (Graham *et al.*, 1994; WHO, 1991; US General Accounting Office, 1990) – guidelines will be developed for treatment evaluation which can be used not only for self-evaluation, but also for comparative evaluation of different treatments. Training courses will also be organised for researchers, professionals and administrators providing an introduction to the methodology of self-evaluation, comparative evaluation and the implementation of evaluation results.

International research projects

A number of national research projects and four multi-site international studies have been initiated on the basis of material prepared by COST A-6. These four are:

- The co-morbidity study, which tested the validity of EuropASI through the dual diagnosis of out-patients and those in residential treatment. This study was co-ordinated by the Athens University Mental Health Research Institute, and involved Germany, Greece, Italy and the Netherlands.
- The University of Maastricht has co-ordinated a study aimed at improving psychiatric treatment by preventing relapse in residential programmes for newly dependent drug users. The participating countries were Belgium, France, Germany, Greece, the Netherlands, Italy, Spain and the United Kingdom.
- A Delphi study, co-ordinated by the Ludwig Boltzmann Institut für Suchtforschung in Vienna, aimed at achieving a consensus on the format and content of evaluation in primary prevention. Participants included Austria, Germany, Italy, the Netherlands, Poland, Portugal, Spain and Switzerland.
- At the time of writing, multinational research on cross-border drug-related delinquency, drug tourism and street-level policing was also in preparation.

An extensive report on the Delphi study and a report from the working group on the evaluation of policies are both now available (Springer and Uhl, 1998; Waal, 1998), although the other project reports are still in preparation.

Recent European drug research and future research needs

On behalf of the EMCDDA, the COST A-6 chairpersons have prepared an overview of recent international studies in the fields of epidemiology, drug policy, drug-related delinquency and the evaluation of primary prevention, treatment/rehabilitation and harm-minimisation approaches. They also made recommendations for future research in these fields. The recommendations relevant to treatment evaluation were as follows:

• methods should be defined to enable treatment needs relevant to the development of treatment services to be identified;
• treatment networks in a given territory should be evaluated;
• comparative assessments of cost-effectiveness in treatment should be undertaken;
• the effects and limitations of non-professional interventions should be evaluated;
• treatment accessibility for high-risk groups (deprived youth, refugees, prison inmates, etc.) should be evaluated;
• more research is needed into the reasons for post-treatment relapse; and
• quality standards and quality assurance in substance-abuse treatment need to be developed.

Collaboration with the EMCDDA

Major steps have already been taken by the European Monitoring Centre for Drugs and Drug Addiction to continue the work initiated by COST A-6. The monograph *Evaluating Drug Prevention in the European Union* (EMCDDA, 1998a) and the *Guidelines for the Evaluation of Drug Prevention* (EMCDDA 1998b) have also helped determine how the theoretical work carried out by COST A-6 can be further developed and implemented through the REITOX system.

To this end, a joint workshop was held in Zurich in December 1997, which signified a symbolic 'hand-over' of the work on treatment evaluation from COST A-6 to the EMCDDA.

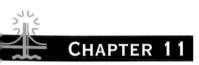

CHAPTER 11

WORLD HEALTH ORGANISATION
PROGRAMME ON SUBSTANCE ABUSE

Maristela Monteiro

From the public-health perspective, it is becoming increasingly evident that substance use plays a major role in morbidity and mortality on a world-wide scale. Despite efforts at controlling the supply of illegal substances and an increase in initiatives for primary prevention, large numbers of individuals are developing harmful or dependent patterns of substance use, leading to disorders requiring treatment.

As defined by the World Health Organisation (WHO), health is 'not only the absence of infirmity, but a state of complete physical, mental and social well-being'. The term 'treatment' should, therefore, be used to define the process that begins when psychoactive substance users come into contact with a health provider or service, and continues through a systematic succession of specific interventions until the highest attainable level of health and well-being is reached. Treatment thus includes comprehensive approaches to detection, assistance, health care and the social integration of those people that present problems as a result of psychoactive substance use.

Treatment evaluation

While recognising the great difficulty of conducting properly controlled and valid research in the area of treatment evaluation, the questions of cost and effectiveness can still be investigated and prioritised. This approach would help to ensure the most effective use of available human and financial resources.

To rationalise the allocation of resources for teatment based on evaluation, it is first necessary to educate policy- and decision-makers, as well as programme-managers, in the need for such assessment. An appreciation of the benefits of, and the need for, proper evaluation must be developed before this procedure can be fully accepted and implemented on a regular basis.

Substance-use services can be evaluated on many levels. These levels include the treatment components, services, programmes and systems. At its simplest, evaluation may focus on individual treatment activities or components, such as one-to-one counselling or pharmacotherapy. At the service level, assessment focuses on the individual or on the combined effects of interrelated treatment activities. At the programme level, evaluation focuses on single or multiple treatment services provided by a single administrative entity. Finally at the systems level, the evaluation focuses on the full complement of programmes available either in a defined community, in larger geographic regions or at national level. This chapter looks at each of these levels of evaluation.

Evaluation goals

Treatment evaluation should be seen above all in the context of a society that endeavours to reduce substance-use problems by providing accessible and afford-able treatment services and strives unremittingly to improve their quality and effectiveness, within the constraints of available resources.

Two broad goals have been developed to help guide this vision. The first concerns the overall allocation of resources for treatment services. The second concerns the distribution of these resources across the continuum of services.

- *Goal 1:* the allocation of resources to plan, deliver and evaluate psychoactive-substance-use services should be appropriate to the size of the burden that such substance use is placing on that society and the availability of resources to reduce that burden.
- *Goal 2:* specific types of substance-use service should be planned and delivered on the basis of a careful analysis of needs, competing demands, knowledge of the relative cost-effectiveness of alternative forms of service delivery and the explicit recognition of the scarcity of resources and the need for maximum efficiency in their use.

The World Health Organisation

To achieve these two broad objectives, the aims of the World Health Organisation's project are to:

- increase awareness of the role of evaluation in planning and delivering substance-use services;
- increase knowledge of different types of evaluation, their purposes and limita-tions;
- increase confidence and skills in planning and undertaking evaluation activities, especially outcome and economic evaluations; and
- increase the use of evaluation results to improve decisions about programme enhancement and resource allocation.

Why undertake evaluations?

On a general level, evaluation is concerned with obtaining feedback about the oper-ation, effectiveness and efficiency of a treatment activity, service, programme or system. This feedback can be put to several different uses, and the reasons for a particular evaluation must therefore be made explicit from the outset since this will influence all aspects of its planning, design and conduct.

Most of the reasons for undertaking an evaluation fall into two categories:

- First, many evaluations are undertaken from the perspective of *accountability*. Such studies often set out to judge whether the treatment programme is actually delivering what it has promised, either in terms of the services provided or the outcomes achieved. Accountability evaluations place considerable emphasis on assessing the efficacy or cost-effectiveness of the programme by using rigorous scientific methodologies and are usually conducted by external evaluators in order to bring objectivity to the evaluation process.

- Second, many evaluations are undertaken from a *quality-improvement* perspective. These have the explicit objective of enhancing the service rather than judging its overall worth or accountability. Such studies may examine a wide range of issues related to the cost, delivery and effectiveness of the service.

- Evaluations based on quality improvement are often undertaken with more limited evaluation resources than scientific evaluations, and are usually conducted internally. Increasingly, these internal evaluations take place in a participatory fashion involving, for example, key stakeholders such as managers, treatment staff, community partners and the service's clients themselves.

As well as clarifying the theory that ties together service activities and objectives, evaluation is also undertaken to determine the philosophy and principles underlying the service. Clarification of these principles makes selecting appropriate outcome measures easier. For example, evaluating a service based on harm reduction could focus on broader outcomes than a service based on abstinence.

Discussing people's expectations of the evaluation and their value system, and conducting a systematic review of the programme's logic model greatly facilitates the identification of the key questions and issues that the evaluation should address. These questions and issues should then be prioritised and the details of the evaluation planned. The evaluation assessment culminates with a clear statement of:

- the components of the service to be evaluated;
- the questions to be addressed; and
- the specific data-collection strategies, measures and analyses to be employed.

It also includes a work plan for the evaluation itself.

Needs assessment

There is no universally agreed definition of 'need'. For example, some countries whose national policies do not tolerate any substance use may prevent methadone-maintenance programmes from being implemented. In states where alcohol use is prohibited, controlled drinking is not an achievable goal. Despite the content of national policies, the philosophies of some services may also determine the treatment goals, regardless of the needs of the population to be treated.

Needs assessment usually involves two distinct phases:

- need identification; and
- need prioritisation.

A variety of approaches and data-collection strategies may be used to identify need. Some methods – such as population surveys, focus groups or community fora – collect information directly from community members, while other approaches – such as key informant surveys or the Delphi technique – rely on input from professionals in the field who are thought to be particularly knowledgeable about the needs to be addressed.

Other approaches use statistical indicators to assess the nature and extent of substance-use problems in the community (such as drug-related crime, liver cirrhosis mortality rates, traffic accidents and family breakdown) as direct or indirect measures of community need. Each of these methods has its strengths and limitations and thus a convergent approach using a combination of these procedures is recommended.

The following questions tend to be asked in a needs assessment:

- What is the prevalence and incidence of substance-use disorders in the community?
- What type of treatment intervention should the service provide?
- What are the main gaps in the community treatment system?
- What is the projected demand for treatment in the community?

For needs assessments undertaken at community level, it is common practice to conceptualise an ideal continuum of services and then to use this as a template with which to assess the availability and accessibility of local or regional services. Estimates of the anticipated demand and the resource requirements for a specific treatment service may also be derived.

It is, however, often difficult to prioritise identified needs because of the political nature of the decision-making process and the lack of clear protocols that reduce bias. If the task is to prioritise which geographic area has the highest need, it may be possible to develop composite indices of various need indicators and then use the ranking of this index to prioritise the various areas under consideration. If, on the other hand, the task is to select the highest priority among a range of service options, then a structured decision-making approach such as a Multi-Attribute Utility Analysis could be used to achieve group consensus and reduce bias.

Costing frameworks

The broad aim of costing studies is to trace the resources used under different circumstances. There are three main ways in which costs could be addressed:

- by estimating the social cost to the community of substance-use problems;
- by undertaking cost-minimisation studies, which compare the costs of alternative treatments where outcomes are assumed to be equivalent; and
- by using treatment-resource tracing, which produces a detailed analysis of the different costs involved in delivering a service with an emphasis on how costs may change in relation to activity levels within the service.

Social costs

Social-cost studies trace the impact of a particular substance within a specific location in an allotted time period. Information on the burden that a particular substance places on a society helps to guide policy action. The disadvantage of such studies is that they do not in themselves evaluate alternative policies which may reduce this burden.

Cost-minimisation studies

In a cost-minimisation study, the resources needed to deliver different treatments are calculated and compared. If outcomes are found to be equivalent, it may suggest that the treatment that required the least resources should be considered further. In most cost-minimisation studies, only the direct resources concerned in delivering care are compared. However, since people with substance-use problems use more health and welfare services than people without such problems, the expected resource needs across the whole range of health and social welfare services should be considered.

These studies may be used as a preliminary check on the feasibility of treatment options prior to a more detailed outcome or economic evaluation. If there is firm evidence to suggest that there would be no difference in outcomes across the many domains considered, a cost-minimisation comparison could be seen as a form of economic evaluation.

Treatment-resource tracing

These studies are designed to examine the costs of the resources required to deliver specific units of service (such as counselling sessions). The information from such research can be used by providers to set their charges and monitor whether resources are being used as planned. For such evaluations, it is important to distinguish between fixed costs and semi-fixed costs.

Outcome evaluation

The two tasks of treatment-outcome research are:

- to measure change associated with treatment; and
- to infer causality.

A number of evaluation designs allow these two tasks to be achieved to varying degrees.

Design models

As discussed in earlier chapters, the most widely praised design in terms of measuring change and inferring causality is the randomised control trial, wherein patients are randomly assigned to receive one of two or more treatment options. From the scientific point of view, such trials are considered the 'gold standard' in evaluating treatment effects, because the design allows for the inference of causality, and changes may be more easily attributed to the treatment examined rather than to other extraneous factors.

Another design model, which is still relatively robust in its ability to allow causal inference, is the 'quasi-experimental' approach, wherein patients are not randomly assigned to treatment. Rather, two groups of patients which have received two different treatments are compared. In this design, the ability to make strong inferences of causality is improved if patients in the two treatments are matched or if pre-treatment differences are adjusted statistically. If such a matching or statistical adjustment does not take place, it is possible that any variations which favoured one treatment over the other were due to factors that presented prior to the start of treatment.

Nonetheless, even a two-group comparison without matching or adjustment is more useful in determining the relative effectiveness of treatment than a single-group design. These studies simply analyse the progress of a group of patients over time and do not allow any inferences to be made about relative effectiveness. Patients are monitored in terms of changes from pre- to post-treatment, and these changes are directly attributed to the treatment provided. The strength of this inference, however, is quite weak because patients may improve simply because of the passage of time or as a result of other unrelated factors.

The weakest method of determining causation is the single-group study where patients are assessed only at the end of treatment. Although the clinician may have faith that the patients have improved, with no measure of pre-treatment problems it is impossible to draw conclusions about the extent of change and its relationship to the provision of treatment.

Whatever evaluation design is selected, the issue remains of which outcomes will be measured and how. Measures should be reliable, scientifically valid and appropriate to the interventions' objectives. This means that the measures must be sensitive to behavioural change over time, and able to assess the patient's well-being accurately.

A number of domains are typically included when examining outcome:

- substance-use frequency and pattern;
- psychological functioning;
- physical health (including HIV status);
- social adjustment;
- family functioning;
- employment; and
- criminal activity.

It is not, however, always necessary to measure all these factors when evaluating a treatment approach.

Economic evaluation

Economic evaluations can be used to answer different questions. For example, funders, policy-makers or even the general public may require an answer to the question 'is treatment worthwhile and does it result in more benefits than costs?'

Both providers and funders of services may be interested in the answer to questions such as 'which of the treatment options or combinations provides the best value from the budget available?'

A more generally relevant question for publicly funded health and welfare systems concerns the choice of allocating resources to different client groups or types of provider agencies. For example, the question may be asked of how to distribute available resources between treatment services and other types of health-care services.

Economic evaluations require the identification of all costs and benefits for the alternatives under consideration. As already outlined in Chapter 5 above, costs can be direct or indirect, while benefits involve positive changes in the quality of life for the individual, his or her family and society as a whole.

Conclusions

In conclusion, the following recommendations can be made:

- that governments and policy-makers encourage and support the standardised evaluation of treatment approaches to substance-use disorders;
- that governments use results from evaluations of cost-effectiveness when planning national treatment services in order to allocate resources more efficiently;
- that governments use concepts of equity in providing accessibility to treatment;
- that governments in all WHO Member States plan national treatment systems taking into consideration local evaluations of effectiveness and the economic efficiency of different treatment approaches;

- that the WHO Programme on Substance Abuse co-ordinates the production and testing of guidelines on treatment evaluation to be used by programme-managers and administrators; and
- that programme-managers and administrators plan, develop and implement activities, programmes, services and systems to evaluate treatment, and use the information gathered from them to improve the cost-effectiveness of treatment provision.

WORKSHOP CONCLUSIONS

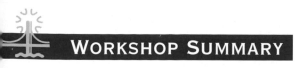

PART IV

Anna Kokkevi

The need for treatment evaluation

Given both the growth in drug-related problems and the limited resources that can be dedicated to reducing them in a period of economic constraint, the need properly to manage the cost-effectiveness of treatment and to ensure the highest quality and best outcomes for the lowest possible cost are indisputable priorities.

In Europe, drug-treatment evaluation research has been mainly limited to small-scale clinical studies. The UK's National Treatment Outcome Research Study (NTORS) is one of the exceptions to this rule, being probably the first large-scale, nationwide attempt to evaluate drug treatments in Europe.

A multi-centre European study, carried out in five countries and entitled Psychosocial Problems and Psychiatric Co-morbidity among Drug and Alcohol Dependent Persons applying for Treatment, also includes a number of evaluation parameters and standardised assessment instruments. However, it must again be emphasised that such studies are rare and so, to date, much of the discussion about measuring treatment effectiveness has centred on academic debate.

The effectiveness of drug treatment

Three positions in this debate were presented during the workshop.

*   *The nihilistic position* questions whether the right to treatment and care, based on ethical standards of medicine, is a sufficient basis for allocating scarce resources. If   as has been claimed by some – treating problematic drug users produces poor results at best, then not only treatment development, but also the allocation of funds need to be reconsidered. If, on the other hand, treatment is seen to mitigate drug-related problems, evidence must be provided for this based on valid and reliable data.

    In support of the argument for evidence-based treatment, Mats Fridell sought to clarify the traditional misconception of the high 'spontaneous remission' of addiction. This concept could lead to the false and even dangerous belief that treatment is of limited value, as the individuals undergoing it would have recovered anyway. Spontaneous remission at rates of 50%, as reported by some studies, would seem to indicate that treatment is in fact not worthwhile. In such a case it could be argued that spontaneous remission is less costly than treatment.

However, well-documented studies reviewed by Fridell show that spontaneous remission is actually in the range of 10–15%. This illustrates the methodological pitfalls that can lead to false claims about the effectiveness or otherwise of treatment. In his presentation, Fridell stressed the need to apply appropriate methodology to satisfy valid treatment-outcome evaluation.

- *The utopian position* faces many of the same problems as the previous one. Vincent Hendriks referred to studies that reported treatment effectiveness at levels of 80% and above. He argued that such studies are in reality boosting their results by applying evaluation approaches designed to cope with pressure from funding organisations and to satisfy expectations, rather than ensuring evaluation validity.

- *The realistic position* was posed by both Fridell and Hendriks. The current position – according to Hendriks' literature review – seems to follow the 'rule of thirds': one-third of clients achieve abstinence; one-third improve, but are not abstinent; and one-third make no progress.

A recently completed Swedish study reported by Fridell found that at five-year follow-up, 40% of heavy drug abusers who had undergone detoxification or short-term rehabilitation had been abstinent for two years. There was also an overall decrease in all forms of drug consumption and a significant reduction in criminal activity. Fridell also cited a recent UK overview which concluded that success rates for the treatment of substance disorders are as high or higher than those for many other chronic ailments, and that any critical appraisal of the effects of drug treatment must include comparisons with other types of treatment for other medical conditions.

Evi Hatziandreou also pointed out that the (albeit limited) number of available studies suggest that the benefits of treatment seem to be at least as great as its costs.

Concepts used in evaluation research

Mats Fridell clarified and distinguished the concepts most frequently applied in evaluation research as follows:

- *productivity*   the relationship between achievements and resources;
- *effect*   the relative difference between two treatment methods or a specific treatment method and control groups that receive an alternative treatment or placebo;
- *effectiveness*   the relationship between effects and resources;
- *efficacy*   the measurement of the relative scale of an effect in a treatment meta-analysis;
- *treatment outcome*   a concept deemed to be more appropriate and precise than either 'effect' or 'efficacy' when evaluating residential treatment.

Evi Hatziandreou further clarified the basic concepts used in economic evaluation research:

- *cost–benefit*   the ratio between the costs and benefits – both measured in monetary terms – that arise from a particular treatment intervention;

- *cost-effectiveness*   the ratio between the costs and benefits that arise from a particular intervention, where benefits are calculated in 'health' and 'social' rather than in monetary terms;

- *direct costs*   the measurement of the value of resources consumed (both health- and non-health-related);

- *indirect costs*   the measurement of the value of lost productivity;

- *intangible costs*   the measurement of costs relating to the isolation, stress, pain and suffering of those afflicted by substance abuse.

Meeting the needs of the practitioner

Heinrich Küfner pointed out that clinicians and practitioners are more interested in the evaluation of single treatment components than the overall evaluation of treatment. It is rare for evaluations to provide an indication as to 'what works', although estimates of cost and evidence of the benefits of individualised approaches can be made.

Küfner also stated that evaluation results have a limited influence on the treatment system. He explained this situation both in terms of the problems and the limitations inherent in evaluation research and of the shortcomings of some clinicians.

In reality, social trends have more influence on treatment directions than do the results of evaluation studies. But, despite the neglect or under-use of evaluation results and the problems encountered, Küfner felt that there is no alternative to evaluation.

He further underlined the need for a close relationship between researcher and clinician. This collaboration can lead to the identification of clinically significant evaluation criteria.

Meeting the needs of the policy-maker

Elfriede Koller presented the point of view of the policy-maker regarding what is expected from treatment evaluation. Treatment effectiveness needs to be proved by means other than 'face validity' criteria, and policy-makers need to know how input (money) and outcome (socially integrated clients) are balanced.

Policy-makers also require information on the comparative effectiveness of different treatment approaches. This will help in planning treatment more effectively, as well as in assessing the care system as an integrated entity, rather than focusing on a specific institution or programme. Ultimately, policy-makers want to be able to identify gaps in inter-sectoral co-operation and help improve this co-operation to ensure better co-ordination.

This last point was also approached in economic terms by Evi Hatziandreou. She introduced the notion of opportunity cost (the value of the best alternative which is foregone) and further clarified that the real cost of any programme cannot be judged in budgetary terms, but rather by the health and social outcomes that have not been achieved elsewhere. The objective for a society should be to maximise the total benefits to its members.

Methodological designs for treatment evaluation

A central issue in designing evaluation research is that of the *representativeness* of client samples. Representativeness is a prerequisite for the generalisation of findings. Issues relating to methodological designs were discussed in the contributions from Vincent Hendriks, Mats Fridell and Fabio Mariani.

Although the randomised control design is the design of choice for yielding valid results on treatment outcome, there are practical and ethical constraints within the drug-treatment sector on randomising clients into treatment and non-treatment conditions.

Naturalistic studies, comparing pre- and post-treatment, are the most typical evaluation studies carried out. But a number of confounding variables can be expected to influence the treatment outcome in non-randomised designs, thus limiting the validity of conclusions on treatment effect.

Problems related both to randomisation and to its lack were discussed by Hendriks, who concluded that both research designs may seriously threaten the validity of outcome results in naturalistic settings. He advocated opting for two alternative approaches instead:

* to apply non-randomised designs that provide an opportunity to compensate for the loss of 'power' of the randomised approach; or
* to restrict randomisation to specific components within the treatment programme.

It should also be noted that high drop-out levels might distort the interpretation of evaluation results, and they should consequently be considered carefully in designing evaluation research. In his presentation, Mariani proposed a method for dealing with this problem.

Evaluation criteria

Almost all the contributors underlined the need for clearly defined evaluation criteria, as well as the need to use standardised instruments for their assessment. To do so requires models and hypotheses describing the main factors contributing to treatment.

Küfner proposed investing more effort in developing multi-factoral theoretical models to account for the process of ending addiction, such as path analysis as applied to the development of addiction. These models should be closely related to empirical investigations and could be based on systems theory.

Hendriks proposed the following general regression model

$$outcome = constant + client + treatment + process + error$$

where treatment outcome is considered as a function of a constant (people can change without treatment), a variety of client, treatment and process characteristics and an error component. To follow this model, the *client, treatment* and *process* variables need to be assessed appropriately, while complex multivariate regression techniques should be applied to obtain valid results.

Mats Fridell discussed the issue of single or multiple criteria. Empirical research supports the use of multiple criteria, but it should be remembered that the goal should not be unrealistic. He used the SWEDATE project (Berglund *et al.*, 1991) as an example: by using cumulative criteria, the level of success from a follow-up study dropped from 50% when only the criterion of abstinence from drugs was considered, to 10–14% when a full set of criteria of a completely rehabilitated individual was taken into account instead.

Evaluation instruments

Standardised instruments for recording client characteristics have been developed for the multidimensional assessment of functioning in various life areas. Most of the contributors referred to the Addiction Severity Index (ASI) and to its European adaptation (EuropASI). The group discussed the Opiate Treatment Index (OTI), a more recently developed instrument along the same lines as the ASI, as well as the Maudsley Addiction Profile (MAP), which was developed as an assessment instrument for the UK National Treatment Outcome Research Study (NTORS – see Chapter 8).

Mats Fridell provided information on standardised instruments that could be used in parallel with multidimensional screening instruments like ASI to assess co-morbidity in substance abuse.

Self-rating scales, such as the Symptom Checklist 90 (SCL-90), and personality inventories, such as the Minnesota Multiphasic Personality Inventory (MMPI) or the Eysenck Personality Inventory (EPI), are widely used, while structured clinical interviews, such as the Composite International Diagnostic Interview (CIDI), are also available for the assessment of *Diagnostic and Statistical Manual* (DSM) and International Classification of Diseases (ICD) diagnostic classifications. Fridell also referred to a seemingly promising scale, the Individual Schedule for Social

Integration, that has been developed to assess the social network of drug-using patients.

Hendriks underlined the need to improve the quality of instruments or to widen the range of client variables in order to reduce the high level of unexplained outcome variance. He supported the view that in addition to treatment-independent variables, treatment-dependent client variables (such as motivation for treatment and client expectations) should be collected.

Three areas should be considered for instrument development:

- the client's preference for a certain type of treatment;
- the client's addiction model; and
- the client's stage of change.

Treatment factors

As Hendriks pointed out, progress made in quantifying what happens during treatment, both from the client's perspective and that of the treatment, is very limited. Treatment still remains very much a 'black box'. Neither treatment as a whole, nor the interventions within treatment, are well described and understood.

The most frequently studied variables are the intermediate variable of time in treatment and the simple description of the type of treatment under investigation. Hendriks underlined, however, that increased duration of treatment should not be confused with the amount and quality of treatment received.

Fridell emphasised the importance of measuring the 'therapeutic climate' when evaluating organisations and residential treatment. The rationale is that factors like 'climate' and 'culture' are aggregates of organisational dimensions reflecting the selection of patients, the quality and competence of staff members, work satisfaction, conflict levels and organisational structures. The most popular instrument of assessment in this domain is the Ward Atmosphere Scale (WAS) which has been widely used in Scandinavian studies.

Fridell recommended involving staff in a continuous, quality-assurance assessment. However, evaluation by external researchers will be necessary to obtain more reliable information on the long-term effectiveness of various treatment modalities.

Economic evaluation

The various approaches to economic evaluation in the broader health domain apply several common methods:

- measuring costs only;
- measuring both costs and health or social consequences; and
- measuring health-related quality of life.

Evi Hatziandreou briefly described these three methods. She further stated that in the field of drug misuse, economic evaluation has rarely been applied in a systematic and rigorous way. In the past, studies seem to have underestimated the true burden on society by failing to consider certain tangible costs that extend to the drug user, the environment and to society at large.

There is still a lack of rigour in cost–benefit and cost-effectiveness analyses. Progress is, however, being made, and time-series and modelling techniques have been developed to help assess the impact of treatment. Yet, effectiveness still remains more difficult to assess than cost and, so far, there is no straightforward evidence as to whether drug-treatment programmes are cost-effective.

Several methodological obstacles still need to be overcome in the field of economic evaluation, such as the issue of appropriate experimental design, conceptual definitions, selection of objective criteria, controlling confounding variables, difficulties in measuring and assigning monetary values and generalising evaluation results to untreated populations.

Evaluation in practice

The contributions by Umberto Nizzoli and Michael Gossop provided valuable insights into how treatment evaluation is implemented in Europe.

TedEval

Nizzoli discussed the evolution of a database system and the attitudes of drug workers and their managers towards the need for evaluation. With the organisational reform of the Italian regions, the need to collect information at regional level led to the development of an electronic infrastructure that facilitates the computerisation of client information. A 20-item instrument, TedEval, was constructed, describing the severity of the client's status and covering six main areas.

NTORS

Gossop presented the first results from the NTORS, which aims to provide evidence of the effectiveness of national drug-treatment services. NTORS is a large-scale, multi-site, prospective study of treatment outcome in a cohort of more than 1,100 clients who entered drug-misuse treatment services in England during 1995. The methodological design of the study is naturalistic – causal inference is achieved by comparing pre- and post-treatment outcome measures.

Pre-existing differences in client characteristics, as well as social and environmental differences that might influence outcome across programmes, are precisely measured so that they can be taken into account in identifying factors associated with observed outcomes.

The MAP is a set of structured research interviews developed specifically for the NTORS project. Items in the MAP include:

- detailed measures of drug and alcohol use and risk-taking behaviour;
- physical and psychological health;
- social functioning (relationships, employment, education and training); and
- criminal involvement.

Further measures cover psychological aspects of drug dependence, motivation for treatment and coping strategies. Interviews have been designed to be carried out by staff at treatment agencies and the information needs of the study have been balanced against the burden on staff time of interviewing clients.

Initial results from NTORS show substantial improvements in all target problem behaviours immediately after starting treatment. Specific improvements were noted in the use of heroin and other illicit drugs. Reductions were also noted in injecting, needle sharing and criminal behaviour.

The European and international dimensions

Representatives from COST A-6, the Federation of European Professionals Working in the Field of Drug Abuse (ERIT) and the World Health Organisation (WHO) provided information on initiatives in the field of drug-abuse treatment.

COST A-6

Ambros Uchtenhagen, chairperson of COST A-6, detailed the aims of this programme and, more specifically, the work of its sub-groups which have developed initiatives in the field of treatment evaluation.

The main objectives of the COST A-6 programme are:

- to set up networks of researchers at national and international level;
- to collect, analyse and develop relevant material; and
- to stimulate multi-centre studies related to evaluation research.

In the area of treatment evaluation, two working groups have undertaken important initiatives. These groups have:

- developed instruments for client description (EuropASI) and treatment services – these initiatives were followed by training courses at European level and have also provided material for multi-centre studies;
- reviewed the relevant evaluation studies in a number of European countries and the methodology and instruments used in these studies; and

- built up a network of scientists and professionals engaged in evaluation research across Europe to exchange information, organise workshops and prepare guidelines for treatment evaluation.

The needs identified in the treatment-evaluation field differ according to the professional focus – researchers want outcome evaluation, practitioners want process evaluation, and administrators require cost–benefit analysis. Adequate instruments for conducting process evaluation and cost–benefit analysis for international use still have to be identified and developed, while guidelines for treatment evaluation will soon be defined.

Finally, Uchtenhagen underlined the added value in the field of treatment evaluation of COST A-6 joining forces with the EMCDDA, so that the basic initiatives undertaken by the group could be further developed and promoted within the REITOX system.

ERIT

Umberto Nizzoli is the President of ERIT which represents approximately 5,000 professionals in Europe. The Federation aims to exchange information, compare experiences and spread the culture of evaluation. To this end, ERIT organises seminars and studies the institutional and social conditions in each country in an effort to locate evaluation in a particular context.

Systematic work on existing evaluation of medical, psychological and socio-educational treatments in Europe has been supported by EU funding. Results of this work show that the need for evaluation is strongly felt in Europe and its practice, although irregular, is increasing. However, it is often carried out in limited areas and communication with others is lacking. ERIT has also collected instruments used for evaluation systematically through its network (see ERIT, 1997).

World Health Organisation

The WHO's work in the field of drug-treatment evaluation was presented at the workshop by Maristela Monteiro. A three-year project (initiated in 1996) on the effectiveness of drug treatment will develop, test and disseminate international guidelines on treatment evaluation. A training package is being prepared that will be field tested in all WHO regions.

The report of the project's advisory group was presented by Monteiro at the workshop. This paper included the rationale for undertaking a proper evaluation, exploring evaluation assessment, needs assessment, process evaluation, costing frameworks, client satisfaction and outcome and economic evaluation. The report also included recommendations for improving, supporting and standardising treatment evaluations.

Recommendations

The workshop identified the following priority areas in promoting the evaluation of treatment research in Europe:

- To improve the general methodology of evaluation studies by stimulating inter-disciplinary collaboration.

- To develop structural and causal models for connecting theoretical constructs, measurement variables and results.

- To carry out meta-analyses on the growing volume of empirical results.

- To identify key variables to be used as valid evaluation criteria.

- To develop appropriate measurement instruments, especially in the areas of treat-ment-programme and treatment-process variables.

- To promote qualitative studies.

- To promote the standardisation and adaptation of methods and instruments in each EU Member State.

- To improve and develop techniques for economic evaluation.

- To develop guidelines for conducting evaluation studies, including effectiveness and economic evaluation.

- To promote compatibility in data collection and evaluation within and between countries.

- To promote the dissemination of methods, instruments and evaluation results.

- To promote training in evaluation for different groups of professionals:

    practitioners (to learn the principles of empirical research, better understand evaluation research results and develop empirical questions that can be answered by empirical studies);

    managers, policy- and decision-makers (to learn how to formulate questions for researchers, identify which questions can be answered and which cannot, and learn how to understand and make use of evaluation research results); and

    researchers (to increase expertise in applying high-quality evaluation research, and improve the understanding and application of appropriate statistical methods for analysing evaluation data).

RECOMMENDATIONS

Participants at the workshop underlined the fact that the EMCDDA is in a good position to encourage – through its official channels of information, dissemination and training – national governments and decision-makers, as well as clinicians, researchers and programme-managers, to develop and improve drug-treatment evaluation.

The following proposals for the EMCDDA's mid-term demand-reduction work plan were outlined on the basis of the participants' contributions.

Promoting existing knowledge

1. To prepare and disseminate a short publication in all European languages addressed to a large audience of decision-makers and professionals. This could start the process of building an 'evaluation culture'. Topics could include:

- a synthesis of the existing knowledge about treatment practice in Europe;
- practical issues, such as the key questions that professionals and policy-makers need to have answered, whether these questions can currently be answered, and which could be answered after appropriate evaluation studies; and
- a brief description of the EMCDDA's work in the field of treatment evaluation.

2. To organise a conference on treatment evaluation to promote further evaluation methodology based on solid scientific grounds.

3. To publish the proceedings of that conference.

4. To create a data bank of appropriate instruments for treatment evaluation. As well as describing the instruments themselves, the data bank should include information on translations into other languages, their normalisation on population samples in different countries, their application in different studies, their usefulness appraised through the experience of their application, and so on.

5. To collect information on existing evaluation studies in Europe.

6. To establish a committee of experts to review and evaluate existing studies in the field of treatment evaluation and to synthesise information on good practice.

Promoting scientific research

1. To develop instruments to support process evaluation and their testing in different Member States.

2. To initiate a number of key projects at European level to apply, on a pilot basis, evaluation research using a common methodological protocol and standardised instruments in the areas of client, programme, process and outcome assessment.

Promoting evaluation studies at Member State and European level

1. To encourage governments and decision-makers to support standardised evaluation and to use results from evaluation to plan treatment services.

2. To encourage and support the co-ordination of treatment-evaluation services by the National Focal Point or another research institution in each Member State.

3. To obtain ministerial support for planning a joint initiative on treatment evaluation to help improve treatment provision across Member States.

4. To develop in close collaboration with the National Focal Points a European policy document for the joint evaluation initiative.

5. To organise a conference at Ministerial level to discuss and adopt the policy document and to specify the desired outcomes to be achieved 5–10 years after its adoption.

In this way, the EMCDDA could play a leading role in monitoring the implementation of national plans, evaluating progress and disseminating results and materials. A common European goal for the provision of quality treatment could lead to measurable improvements in the health of Europe's drug users and the population as a whole.

Since March 1997, when the seminar that forms the subject of this monograph took place, the EMCDDA has taken further steps in the field of treatment evaluation. The Centre is co-operating with the World Health Organisation (WHO) and the United Nations International Drug Control Programme (UNDCP) to field test and distribute a series of workbooks on different aspects of treatment evaluation. These aspects include:

- needs assessment;
- process;
- client satisfaction;
- outcome; and
- economic evaluation.

The EMCDDA is responsible for testing these workbooks within the European Union, while the WHO is responsible for testing them globally. The strategy includes providing direct support in the form of training and advice to selected local projects either interested in or already involved in treatment evaluation. The workbooks will also be distributed to a number of treatment centres that will constitute a control group. The aims of the workbooks are:

- to elicit feed-back from all the participants, whether in the experimental or control groups;
- to compare the results of both groups in terms of training;
- to provide on-going advice on evaluation; and
- to increase the number of evaluation projects sharing the know-how contained on the workbooks.

A first international training workshop took place in Reggio-Emilia, Italy, in June 1998.

The EMCDDA is also supporting the work of the COST A-6 working group on the evaluation of treatment. This group is developing guidelines for the evaluation of treatment which the EMCDDA plans to publish and distribute. The Centre has also launched studies on demand-reduction activities in the criminal-justice system; alternative measures to prison for drug users; outreach work; and substitution treatment. These overviews pay special attention to current evaluation projects and look forward to establishing criteria for evaluating different types of demand-reduction intervention.

Together with the National Focal Points of the REITOX network, and co-ordinated by Greece, the EMCDDA has been developing an instrument to describe the characteristics of treatment services for implementation at EU level. This instrument is the Treatment Unit Form or TUF. Regarding the collection and dissemination of evaluation instruments, the Centre is creating an Internet-based Evaluation

Instrument Bank to facilitate access to evaluation tools in the field of demand reduction and to provide interested clinical and scientific networks with the latest developments in evaluation.

The EMCDDA has played a major role in facilitating information exchange in the areas covered by the above projects, as well as in other domains in which it may become involved in the future. The Centre's main goals have been to help improve the policies and practice of assistance to drug users by promoting a culture of evaluation. To this end, new information technology, above all Internet and e-mail, have proved particularly valuable for the EMCDDA's work.

BIBLIOGRAPHY

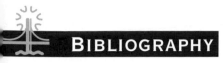

BIBLIOGRAPHY

Apsler, R. (1991) 'Evaluating the cost-effectiveness of drug abuse treatment services' in Cartwright, W., and Kaple, J. (Eds) *Economic Costs, Cost-effectiveness, Financing, and Community-based Drug Treatment*, US Department of Health and Human Services, Research Monograph 113, Washington DC: US Government Printing Office.

Arino, J., *et al.* (1988) 'L'efficacité thérapeutique', *Actes de Vièmes Journées de Reims 'pour une clinique du toxicomane'*, Reims: Centre d'assistance aux toxicomanes (CAST).

Bale, R. N., *et al.* (1980) 'Therapeutic communities versus methadone maintenance – a prospective controlled study of narcotic addiction treatment. Design and follow-up', *Archives of General Psychiatry*, 37, 179–193.

Ball, J., and Ross, A. (1991) *The Effectiveness of Methadone Maintenance Treatment*, New York: Springer.

Bech, P., *et al.* (1986) 'Personality in depression: concordance between clinical assessment and questionnaires', *Acta Psychiatrica Scandinavica*, 74, 263–268.

Bell, M. (1985) 'Three therapeutic communities for drug abusers: differences in treatment environments', *International Journal of the Addictions*, 20, 1523–1531.

Berglund, G., *et al.* (1991) 'The Swedate project: interaction between treatment, client background and outcome in a one year follow-up', *Journal of Substance Abuse Treatment*, 8, 161–169.

Bertling, U., *et al.* (1993) *Substance Abusers with Severe Psychiatric Disorders*, Stockholm: Publica.

Bischof, N. (1995) *Struktur und Bedeutung. Eine Einführung in die Systemtheorie*, Bern: Hans Huber.

Blanken, P., *et al.* (1995) *European Addiction Severity Index – EuropASI. A Guide to Training and Administering EuropASI Interviews*, Brussels: COST A-6.

Brickman, P., *et al.* (1982) 'Models of helping and coping', *American Psychologist*, 37, 368–384.

Cartwright, W., and Kaple, J. (Eds) (1991) *Economic Costs, Cost-effectiveness, Financing, and Community-based Drug Treatment*, US Department of Health and Human Services, Research Monograph 113, Washington DC: US Government Printing Office.

Cázares, A., and Beatty, L. A. (1994) *Scientific Methods for Prevention Intervention Research*, Rockville, MD: National Institute on Drug Abuse.

Cesarec, Z. (1980) 'The Basic Character Trait Inventory – a questionnaire for the measurement of four basic personality traits', unpublished manuscript, Department of Psychiatry and Neurochemistry, University of Lund.

Cesarec, Z., and Fridell, M. (1997) *Some Personality Characteristics in an Inpatient Population of Drug Addicts – Empirical Findings in a Cohort of 202 Hospitalised Drug Addicts*, Lund: University of Lund, Department of Applied Psychology.

Cesarec, Z., and Marke, S. (1968) *CMPS – Cesarec Marke Personality Scheme*, Stockholm: Skandinaviska Testförlaget.

Collins, R., *et al.* (1985) 'Treatment characteristics of psychiatric programs that correlate with patient community adjustment', *Journal of Clinical Psychology*, 41, 299–308.

Colon, I., and Massey, R. (1988) 'Patient attitudes and beliefs as predictors of treatment outcome in detox', *Alcoholism Treatment Quarterly*, 5, 235–244.

Condelli, W., and Hubbard, R. (1994) 'Relationship between time spent in treatment and client outcomes from therapeutic communities', *Journal of Substance Abuse Treatment*, 181, 25–33.

Cook, T., and Cambell, D. (1986) *Quasi-Experimentation – Design and Analysis Issues for Field Settings*, Chicago, Il: Rand McNally College Publications.

Craig, R. (1980) 'Personality characteristics of heroin addicts: a review of the empirical literature with critique II', *International Journal of the Addictions*, 15, 607–626.

Craig, R. (1979) 'Personality characteristics of heroin addicts: a review of the empirical literature with critique I', *International Journal of the Addictions*, 14, 513–532.

Crits-Christoph, P. (1992) 'The efficacy of brief dynamic psychotherapy: a meta-analysis', *American Journal of Psychiatry*, 149, 151–158.

Crits-Christoph, P., and Siqueland, L. (1996) 'Psychosocial treatment for drug abuse – selected review and recommendations for national health care', *Archives of General Psychiatry*, 53, 749–757.

Darke, S., *et al.* (1992) 'Development and validation of a multi-dimensional instrument for assessing outcome of treatment among opiate users: the Opiate Treatment Index', *British Journal of Addiction*, 87, 733–742.

Davidson, R. (1992) 'Prochaska and DiClemente's model of change: A case study?', *British Journal of Addiction*, 87, 821–822.

De Leon, G. (1991) *Retention in Drug-free Therapeutic Communities*, Rockville, MD: National Institute on Drug Abuse.

De Leon, G. (1984) *The Therapeutic Community – Study of Effectiveness*, Rockville, MD: National Institute on Drug Abuse.

De Leon, G., and Jainchill, N. (1986) 'Circumstances, motivation, readiness and suitability as correlates of treatment tenure', *Journal of Psychoactive Drugs*, 18, 203–208.

De Leon, G., *et al.* (1994a) 'Residential drug-abuse treatment research: are conventional control designs appropriate for assessing treatment effectiveness?', *Journal of Psychoactive Drugs*, 27, 85–91.

De Leon, G., *et al.* (1994b) 'Circumstances, motivation, readiness and suitability (the CMRS scales): predicting retention in therapeutic community treatment', *American Journal of Drug and Alcohol Abuse*, 20, 495–515.

Derogatis, L. (1994) *SCL-90-R, Administration, Scoring and Procedure Manual for the Revised Version of the SCL-90*, Minneapolis, MN: National Computer Systems Inc.

Derogatis, L., and Lipman, R. (1973) 'SCL-90: an outpatient psychiatric rating scale – preliminary report', *Psychopathology Bulletin*, 9, 13–28.

Dertell, H. (1989) 'Assessing quality in public service' in Edvardsson, B., and Thomasson, B., (Eds), *Quality Development in Private and Public Service*, Stockholm: Natur och Kultur, 144–163.

Deutsche Gesellschaft für Suchtforschung und Suchttherapie e.V. (1994) *Documentation Standards II for the Treatment of Substance Abuse*, Freiburg: Lambertus.

Drummond, M., *et al.* (1987) *Methods for the Economic Evaluation of Health Care Programmes*, Oxford: Oxford University Press.

Durlake, J., and Lipsey, M. (1991) 'A practitioner's guide to meta-analysis', *American Journal of Community Psychology*, 19, 291–332.

ERIT (1997) *The Evaluation of Medical, Psychological, Socio-educational Interventions with Drug Users in Europe*, Modena: Enrico Mucchi.

European Monitoring Centre for Drugs and Drug Addiction (1998a) *Evaluating Drug Prevention in the European Union*, Scientific Monograph No. 2, Lisbon: EMCDDA.

European Monitoring Centre for Drugs and Drug Addiction (1998b) *Guidelines for the Evaluation of Drug Prevention*, Manuals series No. 1, Lisbon: EMCDDA.

Eysenck, H. (1959) *The Maudsley Personality Inventory*, London: University of London Press.

Eysenck, H., and Eysenck, S. (1964) *Manual of the Eysenck Personality Inventory*, London: University of London Press.

Farkas, A., *et al.* (1996) 'Addiction versus stages of change models in predicting smoking cessation', *Addiction*, 91, 1271–1280.

Fountain, D. (1992) 'Avoiding the quality assurance boondoggle in drug treatment programs through total quality management', *Journal of Substance Abuse Treatment*, 9, 355–364.

French, M., *et al.* (1991) 'Conceptual framework for estimating the social cost of drug abuse', *Journal of Health and Social Policy*, 2.

French, M., *et al.* (1996) 'Estimating the dollar value of health outcomes from drug-abuse interventions', *Medical Care*, 34, 890–910.

Fridell, M. (1996a) *Residential Treatment of Substance Abuse – Organisation, Ideology and Outcome*, Stockholm: Natur och Kultur.

Fridell, M. (1996b) *Psychiatric Disorders and Drug Abuse*, Stockholm: Swedish Council of Social Welfare.

Fridell, M. (1991) *Personality and Substance Abuse – An Integrated Approach*, Swedish Council for Information on Alcohol and Other Drugs (CAN), Report No. 10, Stockholm: CAN.

Fridell, M. (1990) *Quality Management in Psychiatric Drug Abuse Treatment – Effects on Staff and Patients*, Stockholm: Almqvist and Wiksell International.

Fridell, M., Cesarec, Z., and Johnsson Fridell, E. (1996) *Factors Influencing Treatment Outcome in a Short- and a Long-term Perspective*, Lund: University of Lund.

Friedman, A., and Utada, A. (1989) 'A method for diagnosing and planning the treatment of adolescent drug abusers (the Adolescent Drug Abuse Diagnosis – ADAD – instrument)', *Journal of Drug Education*, 19, 285–312.

Friis, S. (1986) 'Factors influencing the ward atmosphere', *Acta Psychiatrica Scandinavica*, 73, 600–606.

Gold, M., *et al.* (Eds) (1996) *Cost-Effectiveness in Health and Medicine*, New York: Oxford University Press.

Gossop, M., *et al.* (1997) *The National Treatment Outcome Research Study. Improvements in Substance Use Problems at Six Month Follow-Up*, London: Department of Health.

Gossop, M., *et al.* (1996) *The National Treatment Outcome Research Study. Summary of the Project, the Clients and Preliminary Findings*, London: Department of Health.

Graham, K., *et al.* (1994) *The Evaluation Casebook. Using Evaluation Techniques to Enhance Program Quality in Addictions*, Toronto: Addiction Research Foundation.

Haastrup, S., and Jensen, P. (1988) 'Eleven-year follow-up of 300 young opioid addicts', *Acta Psychiatrica Scandinavica*, 77, 22–26.

Hallstrom, T., *et al.* (1986) 'Psychological factors and risk of ischaemic heart disease and death in women: a twelve-year follow-up of participants in the population study of women in Gothenburg, Sweden', *Journal of Psychosomatic Research*, 30, 451–459.

Hansson, L., *et al.* (1993) 'What is important in psychiatric inpatient care? Quality of care from the patient's perspective', *Quality Assurance in Mental Health Care*, 5, 41–47.

Hare, R., et al. (1991) 'Psychopathy and the DSM-IV criteria for antisocial personality disorder', Journal of Abnormal Psychology, 163, 391–398.

Hartnoll, R. (1994) Drug Treatment Reporting Systems and the First Treatment Demand Indicator: Definitive Protocol, Strasbourg: Council of Europe, Pompidou Group.

Henderson, S., et al. (1980) 'Measuring social relationships: the interview schedule for social interaction', Psychological Medicine, 10, 723–734.

Holmlund, U. (1990) 'The experiences of dysmenorrhea and its relationship to personality variables', Acta Psychiatrica Scandinavica, 82,182–187.

Hser, Y., and Anglin, D. (1991) 'Cost-effectiveness of drug abuse treatment: relevant issues and alternative longitudinal modeling approaches' in Cartwright, W., and Kaple, J. (Eds) Economic Costs, Cost-effectiveness, Financing, and Community-based Drug Treatment, US Department of Health and Human Services, Research Monograph 113, Washington DC: US Government Printing Office.

Hubbard, R., et al. (1989) Drug Abuse Treatment: A National Study of Effectiveness, Chapel Hill, NC: University of North Carolina Press.

Kelstrup, A., et al. (1993) 'Satisfaction with care reported by psychiatric inpatients – relationship to diagnosis and medical treatment', Acta Psychiatrica Scandinavica, 83, 374–379.

Kersten, T., et al. (1995) Development and Validation of Decision Tree Models for Matching Clients to Addiction Treatment and Care, Nijmegen: Bureau Blta.

Keso, L., and Salaspuro, M. (1990) 'Inpatient treatment of employed alcoholics: a randomised clinical trial of haezelden-type and traditional treatment', Alcoholism: Clinical and Experimental Research, 14, 584–589.

Kiresuk, T. (1973) 'Goal attainment scaling at a county mental health service', Evaluation, 12–18.

Kiresuk, T., and Sherman, R. (1968) 'Goal attainment scaling. A general method for evaluating comprehensive community mental health programs', Community and Mental Health Journal, 4, 443–453.

Kline, P., and Storey, K. (1977) 'A factor analytic study of the oral character', British Journal of Social and Clinical Psychology, 16, 317–328.

Klinteberg, B., et al. (1992) 'Personality and psychopathy of males with a history of early criminal behaviour', European Journal of Personality, 6, 245–266.

Klinteberg, B., et al. (1986) Self-report Assessment of Personality Traits. Individual Development and Adjustment, Stockholm: Department of Psychology, University of Stockholm.

Kolbey, M. M., and Asghar, K. (1992) *Methodological Issues in Epidemiological, Prevention, and Treatment Research on Drug-Exposed Women and Their Children,* Rockville, MD: National Institute on Drug Abuse.

Kosten, T., *et al.* (1992) 'Concurrent validity of the Addiction Severity Index', *Journal of Nervous and Mental Disease,* 171, 606–610.

Küfner, H. (1998) 'Problems of implementing evaluation in a systemic framework' in COST A6 (Ed.), *Country Reports,* Rome: forthcoming.

Küfner, H. (1996) 'Methodological issues in treatment evaluation', in ITACA (Ed.) *Conference Report: Learn and Change: Balance and Future Perspectives of Intervention on Drugs in Europe. Barcelona,* Barcelona: Imprenta Municipal.

Küfner, H., and Feuerlein, W. (1989) *In-patient Treatment for Alcoholism. A Multi-centre Evaluation Study,* Berlin: Springer.

Liebrand, W., *et al.* (1998) *Computer Modelling of Social Processes,* London: Thousand Oaks; New Delhi: SAGE Publications Ltd.

Luce, B., and Elixhauser, A. (1990) *Standards for Socio-economic Evaluation of Health Care Products and Services,* Berlin: Springer.

Maddux, J., and Desmond, D. (1980) 'New light on the maturing out hypothesis in opioid dependence', *Bulletin of Narcotics,* 32,15–25.

Martin, G. W., *et al.* (1989) 'Methodological issues in the evaluation of treatment of drug dependence', *Addictive Behaviour,* 11, 133–150.

MATCH Research Group (1997) 'Matching alcoholism treatments to client hetero-geneity: Project MATCH post-treatment drinking outcomes', *Journal of the Study of Alcohol,* 58, 7–29.

McCusker, J., *et al.* (1995) 'The effectiveness of alternative planned durations of res-idential drug abuse treatment', *American Journal of Public Health,* 85, 1426–1429.

McLellan, A., and Alterman, A. (1991) 'Patient–treatment matching: a conceptual and methodological review with suggestions for future research' in Pickens, R., Leukefeld, C., and Schuster, C. (Eds) *Improving Drug Abuse Treatment,* Washington DC: US Government Printing Office.

McLellan, A., *et al.* (1993) 'Private substance abuse treatment: are some pro-grams more effective than others?', *Journal of Substance Abuse Treatment,* 10, 243–254.

McLellan, A., *et al.* (1992) 'The fifth edition of the Addiction Severity Index', *Journal of Substance Abuse Treatment,* 9, 199–214.

McLellan, A., *et al.* (1983) 'Increased effectiveness of substance abuse treatment – a prospective study of patient–treatment "matching"', *Journal of Nervous and Mental Disease,* 171, 597–605.

McLellan, A., et al. (1985) 'New data from the Addiction Severity Index: reliability and validity in three centers', Journal of Nervous and Mental Disease, 173, 412–423.

McLellan, A., et al. (1980) 'An improved evaluation instrument for substance abuse patients. The Addiction Severity Index', Journal of Nervous and Mental Disease, 168, 26–33.

Miller, W. (1989) 'Matching individuals with interventions' in Hester, R., and Miller, W. (Eds) Handbook of Alcoholism Treatment Approaches: Effective Alternatives, Boston, MA: Allyn and Bacon.

Miller, W., et al. (1993) 'Enhancing motivation for change in problem drinking: a controlled comparison of two therapist styles', Journal of Consulting and Clinical Psychology, 61, 455–461.

Miller, W., and Sanchez-Craig, M. (1996) 'How to have a high success rate in treatment: advice for evaluators of alcoholism programmes', Addiction, 91, 779–785.

Miller, W., and Tonigan, J. (1996) 'Assessing drinkers' motivations for change: the Stages of Change Readiness and Treatment Eagerness Scale (Socrates)', Psychology of Addictive Behaviors, 10, 81–89.

Miller, W., et al. (1995) 'What works? A methodological analysis of the alcohol treatment outcome literature' in Hester, R., and Miller, W. (Eds) Handbook of Alcoholism Treatment Approaches. Effective Alternatives, Boston, MA: Allyn and Bacon.

Moos, R., and Houts, P. (1968) 'Assessment of social atmospheres of psychiatric wards', Journal of Abnormal Psychology, 73, 595–604.

O'Brien, C. (1996) 'Recent developments in the pharmacotherapy of substance abuse', Journal of Consulting and Clinical Psychology, 64, 677–686.

O'Brien, C., and McLellan, A. (1996) 'Myths about the treatment of addiction', The Lancet, 347, 237–240.

O'Connor, E., et al. (1996) 'Gender and smoking cessation: a factor structure comparison of processes of change', Journal of Consulting and Clinical Psychology, 64, 130–138.

Orth-Gomér, K., and Johnson, J. (1987) 'Social network interaction and mortality – a six-year follow-up study of a random sample of the Swedish population', Journal of Chronic Disease, 40, 949–957.

Plotnick, R. (1994) 'Applying benefit–cost analysis to substance use prevention programs', International Journal of the Addictions, 29, 339–359.

Prendergast, M., Podus, D., and Chang, E. (1998) 'Drug abuse treatment effectiveness: a meta-analysis of treatment-control group designs', paper presented at the 60th Annual Scientific Meeting of the College on Problems of Drug Dependence, Scottsdale, AZ.

President's Commission on Model State Drug Laws (1993) *Socioeconomic Evaluations of Addiction Treatment,* Piscataway, NJ: Rutgers University Center of Alcohol Studies.

Prochaska, J., and DiClemente, C. (1983) 'Stages and processes of self-change and smoking: towards a more integrative model of change', *Journal of Consulting and Clinical Psychology,* 51, 390–395.

Prochaska, J., and Velicer, W. (1996) 'On models, methods and premature conclusions', *Addiction,* 91, 1281–1283.

Prochaska, J., *et al.* (1988) 'Measuring processes of change: applications to the cessation of smoking', *Journal of Consulting and Clinical Psychology,* 56, 520–528.

Ravndal, E. (1995) *Drug Abuse, Psychopathology and Treatment in a Hierarchical Therapeutic Community: A Prospective Study,* Oslo: Department of Behavioural Sciences in Medicine, University of Oslo.

Ravndal, E., and Vaglum, P. (1992) 'Different intake procedures – the influence of treatment start and treatment response: a quasi-experimental study', *Journal of Substance Abuse Treatment,* 9, 53–58.

Rice, D., *et al.* (1991) 'Economic costs of drug abuse', in Cartwright, W., and Kaple, J. (Eds) *Economic Costs, Cost-effectiveness, Financing, and Community-based Drug Treatment,* US Department of Health and Human Services, Research Monograph 113, Washington DC: US Government Printing Office.

Roch, I., *et al.* (1992) 'Empirische Ergebnisse zum Therapieabbruch bei Drogenabhängigen. Ein Literaturuberblick', *Sucht,* 38, 305–322.

Sanchez-Craig, M. (1980) 'Random assignment to abstinence or controlled drinking in a cognitive behavioral programme: short-term effects on drinking behavior', *Addictive Behaviors,* 5, 33–39.

Sandell, R. (1994) 'Diagnosing the personality organisation of drug abusers by rating ego balance', *Acta Psychiatrica Scandinavica,* 89, 433–440.

Sandell, R., and Bertling, U. (1996) 'Levels of personality organisation and psychopathology among drug abusers in Sweden', *Journal of Clinical Psychology,* 52, 711–722.

Sandler, J., and Hazari, A. (1960) 'The "obsessional": on the psychological classification of obsessional character traits and symptoms', *British Journal of Medical Psychology,* 33, 113–122.

Simpson, D., and Sells, S. (1990) *Opioid Addiction and Treatment: A 12-Year Follow-Up,* Malabar: Keiger.

Skodol, A., *et al.* (1988) 'Validating structured DSM-III-R personality disorder assessments with longitudinal data', *American Journal of Psychiatry,* 145, 1297–1299.

Skre, I., et al. (1991) 'High inter-reliability for the structured clinical interview for DSM-III-R, Axis I (SCID-I)', Acta Psychiatrica Scandinavica, 84, 167–173.

Smith, M., et al. (1980) The Benefits of Psychotherapy, Baltimore, MD: Johns Hopkins University Press.

Snow, M. (1973) 'Maturing out of narcotic addiction in New York City', International Journal of the Addictions, 8, 921–938.

Springer, A., and Uhl, A. (Eds.) (1998) Evaluation Research in Regard to Primary Prevention of Drug Abuse, Brussels: European Commission.

Süß, H.-M. (1995) 'Zur Wirksamkeit der Therapie bei Alkoholabhängigen: Ergebnisse einer Meta-Analyse', Psychologische Rundschau, 46, 248–266.

Taylor, C., and Young, P. (1997) 'Structural equations and path analysis', in EMCDDA (Ed.), Study of the Options to Develop Dynamic Models of Drug Use and Related Problems Using Epidemiological Data, Lisbon: EMCDDA.

Thornton, C., et al. (1977) 'Voluntary versus involuntary abstinence in the treatment of alcoholics', Journal of Studies on Alcohol, 38, 1740–1748.

Undén, A., and Orth-Gomér, K. (1989) 'Development of a social support instrument for use in population surveys', Social Science Medicine, 29, 1387–1392.

Undén, A., and Orth-Gomér, K. (1984) Social Support and Health. Development of a Survey Method to Measure Social Support in Population Studies, Stress Research Report No. 178:2, Stockholm: Karolinska Institute.

United States General Accounting Office (1990) Case Study Evaluations, Washington DC: General Accounting Office.

Vaglum, P. (1979) Unge Stoffmissbrukere i et terapeutisk Samfunn, Oslo: Universitetsforlaget.

Velicer, W., et al. (1995) 'An empirical typology of subjects within stage of change', Addictive Behaviors, 20, 299–320.

Vogt, M., et al. (1995) 'Ergebnisse zum Modellprojekt Betreung von Drogenabhängigen in bäurlichen Familien' in Institut für Therapieforschung (Ed.), IFT–Berichte, Munich: IFT.

Vuori, H. (1991) 'Patient satisfaction – does it matter?', Quality Assurance in Health Care, 3, 183–189.

Waal, H. (Ed.) (1998) Patterns in the European Drug Scene. An Exploration of Differences, Oslo: National Institute for Alcohol and Drug Research.

Wells, E., et al. (1988) 'Choosing drug measures for treatment outcome studies. The influence of measurement approach on treatment results', International Journal of the Addictions, 23, 851–873.

Winnick, C. (1964) 'The life-cycle of the narcotic addict and of addiction', *Bulletin of Narcotics*, 16, 1–11.

Winnick, C. (1962) 'Maturing out of narcotic addiction', *Bulletin of Narcotics*, 14, 1–7.

Woody, G., *et al.* (1987) 'Twelve-month follow-up of psychotherapy for opiate dependence', *American Journal of Psychiatry*, 144, 590–596.

World Health Organisation (1997) *Evaluation of Psychoactive Use Disorder Treatment*, WHO Workbooks on Evaluation of Treatment (draft).

World Health Organisation (1991) *Evaluation of Methods for the Treatment of Mental Disorders. Report of a WHO Scientific Group*, Technical Report Series 812, Geneva: WHO.

CONTRIBUTORS

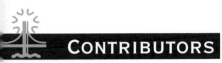

CONTRIBUTORS

Professor Mats Fridell
Department of Applied Psychology
Paradisgatan 5: Ing. 0
S-223 50 Lund
Sweden
Tel: +46-46-222 3321
Fax: +46-46-222 9112

Dr Michael Gossop
National Addiction Centre
4 Windsor Walk
London SE5 8AF
UK
Tel: +44-171-919 3822
Fax: +44-181-776 2026

Ms Evi Hatziandreou
Astra Hellas A.E.
4 Theotokopoulou and Astronafton Street
Maroussi 151 25
Athens
Greece
Tel: +30-1-684 7977
Fax: +30-1-684 7968

Dr Vincent Hendriks
IVO-Institute for Addiction Research
Essenlaan 4
3062 NM Rotterdam
The Netherlands
Tel: +31-10-425 3366
Fax: +31-10-276 3988

Dr Elfriede Koller
Drogenbeauftragte Senatsverwaltung
für Jungend und Familie
Am Karlsbad 8–10
D-10815 Berlin
Germany
Tel: +49-30-26 54 25 79
Fax: +49-30-26 54 23 21

Dr Heinrich Küfner
Institut für Therapieforschung
Parzivalstrasse 25

D-80804 Munich
Germany
Tel: +49-89-36 08 04 10
Fax: +49-89-36 08 0 4 19

Dr Fabio Mariani
Department of Epidemiology and Biostatistics
Clinical Physiology Institute
National Research Council
Via Trieste 41
I-56100 Pisa
Italy
Tel: +39-50-502 771
Fax: +39-50-589 038

Dr Umberto Nizzoli
Azienda USL di Reggio Emilia
Servizio per Tossicodipendenti
Via Amendola 2
I-42100 Reggio Emilia
Italy
Tel: +39-522-295 327
Fax: +39-522-295 515

COST A-6

Professor Ambros Uchtenhagen
Institut für Suchtforshung
Konradstrasse 32
CH-8005 Zurich
Switzerland
Tel: +41-1-273 4024
Fax: +41-1-273 4064

EMCDDA

Ms Margareta Nilson
EMCDDA
Rua da Cruz de Santa Apolónia 23–25
P-1149-045 Lisbon
Portugal
Tel: +351-1-811 3007
Fax: +351-1-813 7943

Ms Petra Paula Merino
EMCDDA
Rua da Cruz de Santa Apolónia 23–25
P-1149-045 Lisbon
Portugal
Tel: +351-1-811 3021
Fax: +351-1-813 7943

University Mental Health Research Institute (UMHRI)

Professor Anna Kokkevi
University Mental Health Research Institute
74 Vas Sophias Avenue
Athens 115 28
Greece
Tel: +30-1-653 6902 / 617 0838
Fax: +30-1-653 7273

WHO

Dr Maristela Monteiro
Programme on Substance Abuse
Division of Mental Health and Prevention of Substance Abuse
World Health Organisation
CH-1211 Geneva 27
Switzerland
Tel: +41-22-791 4791
Fax: +41-22-791 0746

NOTES

133

PRACTICAL INFORMATION

Address:
European Monitoring Centre for Drugs and Drug Addiction
Rua da Cruz de Santa Apolónia 23–25
P-1149-045 Lisbon, Portugal

Telephone:
351 1 - 811 30 00

Fax:
351 1 - 813 17 11

E-mail:
General: info@emcdda.org or emcdda@reitox.net
Private: firstname.surname@emcdda.org or firstname.surname@reitox.net
http://www.emcdda.org

Printed in Italy

EMCDDA, December 1998

European Monitoring Centre for Drugs and Drug Addiction

Luxembourg: Office for Official Publications of the European Communities

1999 - pp. **136** - 16 x 24 cm

ISBN 92-9168-051-6

Price (excluding VAT) in Luxembourg: ECU 16.50